Chemotherapy & Radiation

FOR

DUMMIES®

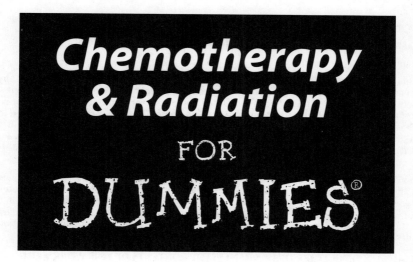

Chemotherapy & Radiation FOR DUMMIES®

by Alan P. Lyss, MD and
Humberto M. Fagundes, MD
with Patricia Corrigan

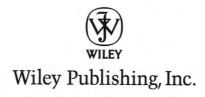

WILEY

Wiley Publishing, Inc.

Chemotherapy & Radiation For Dummies®

Published by
Wiley Publishing, Inc.
111 River St.
Hoboken, NJ 07030-5774
www.wiley.com

For general information on our other products and services, please contact our Customer Care Department within the U.S. at 800-762-2974, outside the U.S. at 317-572-3993, or fax 317-572-4002.

For technical support, please visit www.wiley.com/techsupport.

Wiley also publishes its books in a variety of electronic formats. Some content that appears in print may not be available in electronic books.

Library of Congress Control Number: 2005921459

ISBN-13: 978-0-7645-7832-8

ISBN-10: 0-7645-7832-4

Manufactured in the United States of America

10 9 8 7 6 5 4 3 2 1

1B/QY/QU/QV/IN

WILEY

About the Authors

Alan P. Lyss, MD: Dr. Lyss is the Medical Director of the Missouri Baptist Cancer Center and the Director of the Cancer Research Program of Missouri Baptist Medical Center in St. Louis, Missouri. He is Associate Professor of Clinical Medicine at Washington University School of Medicine and is the honoree of a distinguished Alumni Scholarship Award there. Dr. Lyss also is Associate Clinical Professor at the University of Missouri School of Medicine.

Dr. Lyss is the recipient of several research grants and currently has research funding from the National Cancer Institute. His clinical and research interests are directed toward finding improved treatments for patients with cancer, including improvements in supportive care and psychosocial support. He has been actively engaged in studies directed toward the prevention of common adult cancers and improving the distribution of innovative cancer care to underserved populations, especially to those who reside in rural areas.

Humberto Fagundes, MD: A radiation oncologist, Dr. Fagundes currently holds the position of Medical Director of Radiation Oncology at Missouri Baptist Medical Center in St. Louis, Missouri. He received his training in radiation oncology at Mallinckrodt Institute of Radiology from 1988 through 1992. He was then appointed Chief Resident/Fellow having completed his training in 1993. In the fall of that year he served as Assistant Professor of Radiation Therapy at Loyola University Medical Center in Chicago. Family ties brought him back to the St. Louis area in 1994. In 1999 he arrived at Missouri Baptist Medical Center and was named Medical Director in 2001.

Dr. Fagundes has introduced several innovations at Missouri Baptist, such as 3D Conformal Radiation Therapy, IMRT (Intensity Modulated Radiation Therapy), breast and prostate brachytherapy, as well as intra-operative brachytherapy. His particular interests are in the management of breast and prostate cancers. While in a community hospital, Dr. Fagundes continues to write and publish in the field.

Dr. Fagundes has also worked with the oncology communities in South America and India, where he has assisted in the introduction and implementation of new technologies and cutting-edge treatments in radiation oncology.

Patricia Corrigan: Ms. Corrigan, who holds a B.S. in health education from Lindenwood College, is a reporter for the *St. Louis Post-Dispatch,* where she writes often on health and fitness. She also is the author of 10 books, including *Wild Things: Untold Tales from the First Century at The Saint Louis Zoo* (Virginia Publishing Company), *Convertible Dreams,* a collection of her Post-Dispatch Saturday columns (Virginia Publishing Company), a guide for whale watchers and six nature books for children (NorthWord Press), and a dessert cookbook (Pocketbooks).

Ms. Corrigan has written freelance articles for numerous newspapers across the country and for national magazines such as *More, Ms., BBW, Radiance, Lear's, Family Fun, Cruise Travel,* and *Northwest Travel and Wildlife.* A popular public speaker, she addresses conferences, civic organizations, women's organizations, and school groups. A breast cancer survivor since 1995, she is especially happy to be associated with this book!

Dedication

We dedicate this book to everyone who undergoes chemotherapy and radiation.

Safe trip!

Authors' Acknowledgments

We would like to acknowledge the many cheerleaders in our lives, especially our tolerant families.

Also, for their assistance and unflagging enthusiasm, we also want to thank Jeanne Hanson, Mikal Belicove, Joan Friedman, Ros Hofstein, Jean Roark, Carol Riley, Stephen P. Allen, MD, Gerry Puglisi, Susan Cuddihee, and Linda and Bill Gwyn.

We are grateful for the editorial participation of Martin Raber, MD, clinical professor in GI Medical Oncology at M.D. Anderson Cancer Center in Houston.

Publisher's Acknowledgments

We're proud of this book; please send us your comments through our Dummies online registration form located at www.dummies.com/register/.

Some of the people who helped bring this book to market include the following:

Acquisitions, Editorial, and Media Development

Project Editor: Joan Friedman

Acquisitions Editor: Mikal E. Belicove

Technical Editor: Martin Raber, MD

Editorial Manager: Michelle Hacker

Editorial Supervisor: Carmen Krikorian

Editorial Assistants: Courtney Allen, Nadine Bell

Cover Photos: © Getty Images/Photodisc Collection

Cartoons: Rich Tennant, www.the5thwave.com

Composition

Project Coordinators: Maridee Ennis, Emily Wichlinski

Layout and Graphics: Carl Byers, Andrea Dahl, Joyce Haughey, Stephanie D. Jumper, Barry Offringa

Special Art: Illustrations by Kathryn Born, MA

Proofreaders: Leeann Harney, Jessica Kramer, Carl William Pierce, Dwight Ramsey, TECHBOOKS Production Services

Indexer: TECHBOOKS Production Services

Publishing and Editorial for Consumer Dummies

Diane Graves Steele, Vice President and Publisher, Consumer Dummies

Joyce Pepple, Acquisitions Director, Consumer Dummies

Kristin A. Cocks, Product Development Director, Consumer Dummies

Michael Spring, Vice President and Publisher, Travel

Kelly Regan, Editorial Director, Travel

Publishing for Technology Dummies

Andy Cummings, Vice President and Publisher, Dummies Technology/General User

Composition Services

Gerry Fahey, Vice President of Production Services

Debbie Stailey, Director of Composition Services

Contents at a Glance

Table of Contents

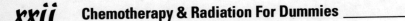

Introduction

You hold in your hands a cancer treatment book with bedside manner.

You can find here facts on chemotherapy and radiation — topics generally perceived as scary, and rightly so — presented in a straightforward manner and a conversational tone. We don't overload you with medical jargon, but we do give you the information you need to have a fruitful conversation with your doctors.

Who are "we"? Fair question. "We" are a medical oncologist, a radiation oncologist, and a professional writer who just happens to be a cancer survivor. Among the three of us, we've accumulated quite a thorough understanding of cancer and its treatments. One of our goals is to provide you with plenty of inside information as you contemplate, begin, traverse, and end your cancer treatments.

Another of our goals is to remind you that even though you spend part of your life as a cancer patient, that part does not define who you are or restrict you as much as you may think.

About This Book

Chemotherapy and radiation are not simple topics, but this is not a dense, academic book. Instead, this is a book written in lay terms with all the material organized in an easy-to-read fashion. We cover one topic at a time in a logical sequence. You may want to start with Chapter 1 and proceed straight through the book in an orderly fashion, or you may want to skip around, reading whatever takes your fancy in any order that you choose.

If your doctor has recommended chemotherapy or radiation therapy, you may want to start with the overview of either, or go straight to a description of what each treatment may mean for you. You decide. Later, if you are curious about some other aspect of these cancer treatments, if you missed something, or if your treatment plan changes, everything you need to know will be waiting for you when you next pick up the book.

Here's another advantage to this book: You can use it to complement the information that your doctors provide. If the details about a specific test, the description of a type of treatment, or a suggestion on how to manage a given side effect eludes you late one night or over the weekend, chances are this book can fill in the blanks until your doctor is back in the office.

Not all cancer treatment guides are created equal. On purpose, this one was developed and written to lead the pack — and to give you exactly the help you need.

Conventions Used in This Book

Some of the material in this book is a little technical and involves some medical terminology. Whenever a new word or phrase is introduced that needs to be defined, the word or phrase appears in *italics* and the definition is close at hand. You may think you don't need to know these words and phrases, but your conversations with your doctors will go more smoothly if you are familiar with the terminology.

Also, all Web addresses in the text appear in a special font, called `monofont`, to set them apart from the rest of the text.

What You Don't Have to Read

Text sitting next to the "Technical Stuff" icon is exactly that. You are welcome to move on if you think you already have plenty of information.

Here's another tip: When you run across any material printed in a gray box, this is material that you may find interesting, but it's not crucial, especially if you are a reader who prefers just the facts about chemotherapy and radiation. Skipping the sidebars will not cause you any trouble in terms of following the rest of the text.

Foolish Assumptions

We have boldly assumed that you are not a medical student, a physician, or a person considering seeking advanced training in oncology or radiation oncology. We also figure you're probably not a contestant preparing for a TV quiz show.

No — we think you have been diagnosed with cancer and are preparing to begin either chemotherapy or radiation, or maybe both. Having cancer ushers you into a whole new world with a whole new language, so we have done our best to explain the culture and define the terms that you are likely to encounter.

On the other hand, you may be shopping for a good reference book to give to a family member or close friend facing cancer treatments. When you hand that person this book, be sure to say we think he or she is lucky to have the support of such a thoughtful person.

How This Book Is Organized

This book is divided into seven parts to help you make your way through cancer treatments.

Part 1: Your Journey Through Cancer Treatments: Preparing for the Trip

This is a suggested packing list, as it were, to ease your experience as you head off to cancer treatments. Here, you find suggestions to help you choose your doctors, a brief refresher course in simple cell biology from your days in science class, and information on some of the tests you may need to schedule to help determine which treatment would be best for you.

Part II: Your Choices along the Way: Making Good Ones

When you have been diagnosed with cancer, you make a lot of important decisions in a short time after you talk with your doctor about which treatments are most likely to stop the cancer. In this part, you get an overview of chemotherapy and radiation therapy — the gold standards today in cancer treatment. Also in this part are many of the answers to questions you may have about clinical trials. And this is where you find detailed information about bone marrow and stem cell transplants.

Part III: Chemotherapy: What to Expect and How to Deal with Side Effects

We can't literally accompany you to your first chemotherapy appointment, but we have been where you are going, and we can tell you what to expect on that day and in the days to come. You've probably heard about the side effects of anticancer drugs. Here, you find them described in detail, one at a time, along with practical suggestions to help you manage those that affect you.

Part IV: Radiation: What to Expect and How to Deal with Side Effects

Preparing to begin radiation therapy? In this part, we take you step by step through your setup appointment, your first dose of radiation, and the remainder of your treatment. This is also the place to look for strategies to help you manage side effects throughout treatments.

Part V: Your Success Strategies: Assembling Your Support Team

We are big fans of the idea of building a support team to call on as you go through cancer treatments. In this part, you find suggestions on how to build good relationships with medical practitioners involved in your care, as well as others you may want to add to the team, including yoga instructors, massage therapists, tai chi practitioners, fitness experts, nutritionists, and spiritual leaders. Here, too, you can decide whether a support group is right for you — and, if so, discover how to find one.

Part VI: Your Future after Cancer Treatments: Looking Ahead

Is there life after cancer? Of course, but don't expect everything to be the same as it was before. In this part, you find an assessment of some of the long-term physical changes that may affect you, a frank discussion on recurrence, and discussions of emotional "potholes" that may exist on the road to your future. You also discover some ideas on how to make the most of every day.

Part VII: The Part of Tens

You've probably heard a lot about cancer, and some of what you heard may even be true! In this part, you discover the real story behind some of the myths of cancer. We also suggest ten specific things people can do to help you as you go through treatment; identify ten matters completely beyond your control; and present what we consider ten gifts from cancer, each of which will make your life after cancer more rewarding. Last of all, look for ten sources for more information about cancer.

Appendix

Cancer comes with its own vocabulary, so look here for a list of words you're likely to hear as you go through cancer treatments.

Icons Used in This Book

Icons used throughout this book call your attention to material that may be of particular use to you.

This is the "helpful hint" icon, and many of the tips provided can save you time and energy, both physical and mental.

How can anybody possibly remember everything there is to know about cancer? This icon serves to remind you of particularly important information.

This icon is intended to set off an alarm — carefully heed any information next to it.

Sometimes, you want to know it all, and sometimes you would just as soon skip the technical stuff. Depending on where you stand, this icon will either flag you down or wave you on.

Where to Go from Here

Our foremost hope is that you go on to live a long and happy life after cancer.

This is your book — take what you need, and may it serve you well.

Part I

Your Journey Through Cancer Treatments: Preparing for the Trip

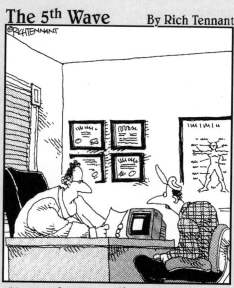

The 5th Wave   By Rich Tennant

"Please Mr. Dugan, I'm an oncologist. I can't be expected to advise you on why your car stalls at stoplights. You'd need to talk to an internist for that."

In this part . . .

Starting with a look at the new world you are entering, we provide tips on what to expect and offer suggestions on how to choose the medical professionals who will accompany you on your journey through cancer treatments. This part also brings you up to speed on what cancer is, how it attacks the body, and what tests are available to help determine the best treatment for you.

Chapter 1

Recognizing the Realities of Chemotherapy and Radiation

. . . .

. . . .

*Y*ou've been told that you have cancer. You may have seen it coming, but more likely this news came out of nowhere to frighten you and shake up your world.

Cancer! How can that be?

Here's how: The Centers for Disease Control reports that more than 18 million new cases of cancer have been diagnosed since 1990, and the government agency estimates that at least 1.3 million new cases will be diagnosed in 2005. One out of every four Americans dies of cancer. In fact, the American Cancer Society announced in January of 2005 that cancer has surpassed heart disease as the leading cause of death for people under 85 in the United States.

On the other hand, more than ever before the words *cancer* and *death* do not necessarily belong in the same sentence. Each day brings news of improvements in screening tests and in treatments. And, happily, survival rates for cancer are at an all-time high in the United States. So, instead of spending time and energy asking "Why me?", we encourage you to take a deep breath and get ready to begin your journey through cancer treatments.

In this chapter, we talk first about taking time to come to grips with your diagnosis. Then we offer suggestions on how to choose a doctor. Next, we present a road map of the rest of this book, where every twist and turn on your journey is clearly marked.

Making Peace with Your Diagnosis

The longest journey begins with a single step, or so an ancient Chinese proverb tells us. You have many steps in store as you make your way through the coming months. But before you take the first step, you have an important task.

Registering your emotions

"First," says one woman we know who was diagnosed with cancer in 1997, "you scream." She is right, even if that scream is silent. This is a logical emotional response. After all, you have never before heard the words, "You have cancer." When you do hear these terrifying words, you may have to ask that the doctor repeat the bad news. Some people recall that on first hearing them, these words sound dim and far away. Others report that their bodies begin to tremble involuntarily. And others appear to remain stonily silent, even as their minds race. Whatever your first reaction, you need time to make peace with your diagnosis.

Taking time to process the news

More likely than not, you won't be thinking clearly at first. You may start to tally up the people you know who have died of cancer, and you probably will wonder if you're going to die, too. At this point, you simply don't have enough information to know what the future holds. You may find yourself totally focused on the diagnosis, but that focus may be chaotic, with hope and fear fighting for your attention even as you try to frame important questions for your doctor.

Give yourself a break. Adjusting to the news that you have cancer takes time. Complete acceptance — if there is such a thing — won't come in a day or a week or even a month, but gradually, you will adjust to the diagnosis. Long before that happens, you may find yourself heading into the operating room for cancer surgery or preparing for your first chemotherapy or radiation appointment. Don't be surprised if, from time to time, you experience the same shock and fear all over again that you felt when you first heard the news.

Experiencing a range of emotions

About that recurring shock and fear: These are completely normal emotions. In fact, you likely will go through repeated periods of denial, anger, bargaining, depression, and acceptance. You may recognize these as the stages that people experience when confronting death. In this instance, you are experiencing the loss of life as you know it, the loss of good health, and the loss of feelings of immortality, so it makes sense that you experience these stages, even if you have treatable cancer.

Expect to take more than one ride on the emotional roller coaster as you move back and forth between a range of feelings. This process definitely involves taking two steps forward and one back.

Over time, you will come to recognize when your emotional well-being is at risk, and you will take comfort in knowing that a period of emotional upset most likely will be followed by a period of calm.

Telling family and friends

Early on, after you have processed the news about your diagnosis and are ready to talk about it, you likely will want to tell family members and close friends so they can make themselves available to provide emotional support — and practical help as well. Many people who are newly diagnosed also want to speak with someone who has had cancer, someone who already has been through treatments and lived to tell the tale. In fact, you may find yourself having an exceptionally keen interest in hearing these tales! If you don't know who to call, you may want to ask your doctor if she can have a survivor get in touch with you.

This is a good time, as you begin to gather information about your diagnosis and potential treatments, to talk with someone who has been there. That said, every individual — for a variety of reasons — experiences cancer and the treatments differently, so remember that the details of someone else's story may not apply to you at all.

You also may want to speak with your boss, as your work schedule and obligations may be directly affected by your treatments. Who else needs to know?

That depends on what type of person you are: The type who needs to tell as many people as possible, or the type who wants to tell as few people as possible. You know yourself best and will act accordingly.

Gathering Information

Knowledge is power! In Part I of this book, we help you get acquainted with the facts about cancer — which actually is more than 100 different diseases — and we describe the tests available to help determine the best treatment for you.

Up until the moment of your diagnosis, you may not have known much about cancer — what it is or how it works (which we discuss in Chapter 2). Now, of course, you want to find out more so you can have an idea about what the coming year holds for you. That's a good, positive approach. A poster passed among people going through cancer treatments reads, "When you know the facts, you can make a plan."

Before you make your plan, your doctor will provide you with specific information about your cancer and recommend appropriate treatments. A number of sources can supply general information, including

- ✔ This book
- ✔ Other books
- ✔ Free booklets published by health agencies
- ✔ Web sites (see Chapter 25 for some recommendations)
- ✔ Newspaper and magazine articles

Some people whip through every bit of reading material available on the type of cancer that they have. Others confine their reading to material that specifically relates to the immediate situation. (We think the latter is a wiser approach.)

You don't have to learn enough to earn a degree in cancer, and you don't have to mold yourself into the perfect patient. Your job is to educate yourself about your specific cancer, get through your treatment, and get on with your life.

Shopping for Cancer Specialists

When we say that it is your job to educate yourself about your cancer and your treatments, please don't think that the responsibility rests entirely on your shoulders. You will have help — a lot of it. Some people first learn that they have cancer from a surgeon or another specialist. When it comes time to do the tests that determine the extent of the cancer — and you can read more about these tests and how to assess your results in Chapter 3 — you need to see a *medical oncologist,* a medical specialist who treats cancer. If radiation therapy is recommended for you, your medical oncologist will refer you to a *radiation oncologist,* a medical specialist who treats cancer patients with radiation therapy.

Finding good doctors

These cancer specialists and other doctors along the way will direct your care and serve as important members of your support team. In Chapter 14, we offer some suggestions for building good relationships with your doctors. Of course, before you can build relationships, you have to choose the doctors. A number of factors come into play, including

- The type of cancer you have
- Your age
- Your general health
- The number of doctors or medical centers available where you live
- Your insurance coverage — or lack of it

Obviously, you want the best care that you can get. Given the state of health-care today, some choices will be up to you and some will not, no matter what your specific circumstances. In any case, you most likely don't want to choose a doctor simply by opening the telephone book and picking one with an office close to your home.

Here are some sources to help you choose your cancer doctors:

- Your primary care doctor (internist or family doctor) or surgeon
- The referral department of a large medical center
- Your local medical society
- Professional medical associations
- A relative or friend who has personal experience with cancer

When you have a name or two in hand, make an appointment for a consultation. Ask the receptionist what you need to do to make any test results, x-rays, or surgical reports available to the doctor. After that information is gathered, sit down with the doctor and hear what he has to say.

If you have a friend or family member who can accompany you for your first visit to the oncologist, take advantage of that help. Another pair of oars could be helpful as you navigate these unfamiliar waters!

Afterwards, think about what you heard. Think about how you felt while you were hearing it. Think about spending the next several months carrying out a treatment plan under the direction of this particular doctor. If you have found a good fit for you, then proceed.

If for any reason you're not satisfied with what you hear, or you are uncomfortable about how you feel, make an appointment with the next doctor on your list.

Second opinions are common in oncology, and most oncologists expect and encourage you to seek one, just so you are comfortable as you proceed with your treatment. A good closing question with the oncologist is "Who would you go to see if you were me and you wanted to be sure that you were on the right path?" If you think that the doctor is uncomfortable with this question, move on!

Preparing to embrace a new culture

After you have chosen a doctor, you quickly will become aware that not only are you in the hands of a new medical professional, but you are entering what may seem like an entirely new culture full of people who speak a new language. (For a crash course in the language, see the glossary in the appendix.) There is much to learn about your particular cancer, of course, but that is just the beginning.

What's next?

- ✔ Tests to take
- ✔ Treatments to undergo
- ✔ Side effects to endure
- ✔ Strategies to implement to manage those side effects

More specifically, just to give you a few examples, you will find yourself wondering about the following:

- ✔ Your blood cell count
- ✔ Survival statistics

- ✔ How radiation works
- ✔ Long-term effects of chemotherapy
- ✔ How to avoid nausea
- ✔ Where to buy a wig
- ✔ Long-term effects of radiation
- ✔ How to care for your skin
- ✔ Clinical trials of new and (potentially) better treatments

And that's just part of your new culture!

Sound confusing? That's why you have this book. We walk you through every step. But first, we have some advice. While you are learning the new language and sorting out your place in the new culture, you also want to keep your eye on the future.

When you have a treatment plan in place, grab a calendar and mark on it the proposed schedule for your chemotherapy and/or radiation treatments. Seeing exactly how long all this will take also allows you to see all those dates left on the calendar *after* treatment, when your life will once again be your own.

Considering Options

Part II of this book is all about options — treatment options, choices regarding delivery of treatments, and the possibility of participating in a clinical trial. Here too you can find complete information on bone marrow and stem cell transplants.

Understanding chemotherapy and radiation

Medical science is currently learning about and testing some ways to turn off the misguided cells that undergo a mutation and get busy transforming into cancer cells that attack the body. Today, chemotherapy and radiation are the time-tested standard treatments for most cancers. Many people diagnosed with cancer have both treatments, sometimes concurrently and sometimes one after the other. Some people have just one.

Basically, most chemotherapy is *systemic;* it involves any number of anti-cancer drugs that sweep through every cell in the body. In contrast, most radiation therapy is *local* or *regional,* meaning treatments are aimed specifically at the site of a tumor or at nearby places the tumor may have spread.

How do these two treatments work? Check out Chapter 4 for details on chemotherapy. We discuss more than half a dozen different types of anti-cancer drugs. Also, though most chemotherapy drugs are delivered directly into a vein, some are injected into a muscle or a tumor. Some chemotherapy drugs even come in pill form. Who knew? Well, if you didn't, see Chapter 4.

Looking for the inside story on radiation therapy? In Chapter 5, you find out about the two main types of radiation therapy — external beam radiation and brachytherapy — as well as some additional types of treatment.

Sometimes your doctors provide you with information and allow you to decide which treatment to pursue. Don't hesitate to ask what choice the doctor would make for a family member, as that may help you with your decision.

In any case, carefully evaluate the benefits and risks of all your treatment options. The decisions you make today may well affect the rest of your life.

Treatments for life-threatening diseases often carry long-term physical costs, such as decreased organ function now or increased risk for other diseases ten years down the road. Paying the price is always easier if you are well-informed before you begin treatments.

Looking into clinical trials

One important option to consider is whether to participate in a clinical trial. These trials, or tests, of new treatments or new combinations of tested treatments lead the way in cancer research. That means the participants in clinical trials are on the cutting edge of medical science. We spell out the pros and cons in Chapter 6, where you also find questions you may want to ask your doctors, as well as reports from participants who have chosen to be part of clinical trials.

Taking a chance on a transplant

Sometimes, in cases where cancer does not respond completely and permanently to standard treatments, doctors recommend bone marrow and stem cell transplants. This is serious stuff, medical miracles of the first order — or so we hear from individuals whose lives have been saved as a result of a transplant. Chapter 7 tells you everything you need to know about the purpose of transplants, the different types, how transplants are done, what to expect afterwards, and how to prepare yourself emotionally.

Exploring Virtual Chemotherapy

There is nothing like the real thing, of course, but in Part III of this book, you come as close to experiencing chemotherapy and all the side effects as you can without actually feeling the powerful anticancer drugs drip into your body.

Getting started on chemo

That first day of chemo, as fearful as it seems in the anticipation, most often doesn't turn out to be as bad as you may expect. In Chapter 8, we take you step by step through your first appointment. In this book, we say repeatedly that you don't have to go through cancer treatments alone. Here, we go so far as to recommend what to eat for breakfast and what to wear! Later in the chapter, we clear up any misconceptions about when to take anti-nausea medication. You also find suggestions on how to get the support you need from family and friends as you go through treatments.

Taking care of your immune system

Because anticancer drugs kill healthy cells as well as diseased cells, you are particularly prone to infection while undergoing chemotherapy. That's bad, because you simply won't have the resources to fight off bacteria that means to do you harm. The good news is that doctors can prescribe immune and bone marrow stimulants to help boost your immune system and help your body fend off infections. In addition to medical interventions, there are plenty of preventative measures that you can take to help protect yourself. Read all about it in Chapter 9.

Signing up for side effects

Even people who have never known anyone diagnosed with cancer seem to know a complete litany of the side effects that accompany this powerful head-to-toe therapy. Never mind that many people taking anticancer drugs are troubled by just a few side effects — and some of those to a limited degree. Everybody wants to get into the act!

In Chapters 10 and 11, you can find details about the serious and not-so-serious side effects of chemotherapy. Here are just some of the side effects we cover:

- ✔ Nausea
- ✔ Fatigue
- ✔ Neuropathy (nerve damage)
- ✔ Mouth and throat sores
- ✔ Depression
- ✔ Infertility
- ✔ Temporary hair loss

Before you panic and assume that you will experience every possible side effect known to result from chemotherapy, we want to say something that we say often in this book, simply because it's comforting to hear.

Every person experiences cancer treatments differently, but no one person is likely to be troubled with every side effect from any one treatment.

No matter which specific side effects you must endure, in this book you find plenty of practical suggestions on how to manage them.

Trying on Radiation Therapy for Size

True to the title of this book, detailed information on what to expect from radiation therapy follows just after we inform you about what to expect from chemotherapy. That's what Part IV is for.

Getting set up for the first treatment

Ask about your first treatment — and in Chapter 12, we answer. You can read all about how radiation therapy is devised specifically for your body. You discover that undressing for the therapy takes longer than the therapy itself. And, we make suggestions about how to care for your skin. If you are looking for ideas on how to get the support you need from family and friends, we provide them here.

Managing side effects

Contrary to popular opinion, people who undergo radiation therapy are every bit as subject to side effects as people who undergo chemotherapy.

Just because Chapter 13 provides details on a long list of side effects, this does not mean that you will experience every last one.

Here are some of the typical side effects from radiation therapy that are described in this chapter:

- ✔ Fatigue
- ✔ Reddened skin
- ✔ Inflamed mucous membranes
- ✔ Diarrhea
- ✔ Nausea
- ✔ Lymphedema (swelling of an arm or leg because of fluid accumulation)
- ✔ Permanent hair loss
- ✔ Depression

We don't simply list possible side effects and then leave you wondering what to do. Plenty of practical suggestions on how to manage those side effects also are included in Chapter 13.

Sending for Help

A recurrent theme in this book is the importance of putting together a support team to help you get through cancer treatments. Some teams are small — tight circles of medical professionals and family members. Other teams may be much larger and include all manner of healthcare professionals, spiritual advisors, and members of support groups. We take a look at all these possibilities in detail in Part V. Regardless of the size of your team or whether you all choose to wear matching T-shirts or baseball caps, having a support team is an important success strategy.

Making room on the team bus

We suggest in Chapter 14 that you let the doctors sit at the front of the team bus, right behind your immediate family and dearest friends. Who comes next? Perhaps a psychologist, if you think you would benefit from that type of help. Next, we propose that you consider looking at a number of complementary therapies that may help you reduce stress as you go through treatments. Practitioners who provide these therapies include

- Massage therapists
- Yoga teachers
- Reiki practitioners
- Tai chi instructors
- Meditation instructors
- Fitness experts

Now, you may be interested in working with only one or two of these individuals — you may not have the time, energy, or funds to take on any more. We encourage you to do that.

Let's face it: Cancer increases stress at both emotional and physical levels. Sometimes, a little body work from a certified practitioner is just what the doctor ordered.

Practicing good nutrition

Both chemotherapy and radiation therapy can cause changes in your eating habits, for a variety of reasons. In some cases, the treatment itself is responsible. In others, fatigue from the treatments can leave you too tired to eat. That's bad, because good nutrition is especially important during cancer treatments. Here are some reasons why:

- Eating well helps you keep your energy up.
- Good nutrition helps you manage side effects.
- A healthy diet can help your body fend off infection.

In Chapter 15, we talk about the importance of good nutrition and even suggest that you may want to add a registered dietitian to your support team.

If you opt not to do that, we make recommendations for a nutritious diet and bring you up to speed on the latest scientific thinking on protein, carbohydrates, fats, vitamins, minerals, and fluids — at least in regard to nutrition during cancer treatments. We also outline for you exactly what nutritional effects specific cancer treatments may have on your body.

Tending to your spirit

Making room in your life for a cancer diagnosis almost always also means asking yourself some of the really big questions — questions most often left to philosophers and spiritual leaders. Some of these questions include

- ✔ Who am I?
- ✔ Why am I here?
- ✔ What is my purpose?
- ✔ Why did I get cancer?
- ✔ Will cancer kill me?
- ✔ What is the point of living in a world where there is cancer?

These questions can lead to a great deal of stress, which can evolve into losing the will to go on or even to a complete loss of faith in the future. This is known as *spiritual distress*.

Who do you call in this situation? In Chapter 16, we talk about faith and make suggestions on how to bring up this topic with your doctors. We also talk about prayer and meditation as ways to reduce spiritual distress. And we recommend that you add a spiritual leader to your support team if you are so inclined.

Finding support from strangers

Sometimes, people going through cancer treatments find that their daily concerns, complaints, and fears may wear out some of the "inner circle" members of the support team. Sometimes, you can find a certain freedom and acceptance from a support group that can't be found anywhere else. Is a support group right for you? Have a look at Chapter 17, where we can help you decide.

In that same chapter, you discover that support can come from many or one, and that you can meet at a hospital, in a church, in a freestanding community center — or in your own home, sitting at your computer. We also review the benefits of being part of a support group, as well as the risks.

Looking Beyond Cancer Treatments

When you're in the middle of chemotherapy or radiation treatments, sometimes it seems that this particular journey will never end. It will, of course, and in Part VI, you discover what to expect when that happens. As at the end of any meaningful road, you're likely to find several forks. In this case, you may want to explore lingering physical side effects of cancer treatments, the possibility of recurrence, and some emotional adjustments that are often required after treatments are complete.

Beginning anew

Don't for a minute expect that you never need darken your doctor's door after the last of your cancer treatments. On the contrary, you will be carefully monitored for years to come. In time, you'll even appreciate that fact.

In Chapter 18, you find out what to expect in terms of follow-up care — regular checkups and periodic screening tests — and you can look over a list of long-term side effects that may or may not trouble you. That list includes such physical problems as the following:

- Fatigue
- Pain
- Lymphedema
- Oral problems
- Bladder and bowel problems
- Early menopause
- Infertility or impotence

Also in Chapter 18, we propose that you craft a personal wellness plan to see you through the years to come.

Returning to square one

Some people finish cancer treatments and never have to confront this particular disease again. In Chapter 19, you get an idea of what to expect if that's not the case — if cancer recurs months or years after treatments end. If you're tempted to avoid this chapter because you expect only the worst, think again.

In many cases, a recurrence can be treated as a flare-up, and cancer can be considered as a chronic disease.

We lay out a plan of action in Chapter 19, should your cancer recur, and we also explain several reasons why the second time around may not be as trying as the first. If recurrence is as bad, or even worse, look here for information on palliative care and an explanation of the mission of hospice.

Making peace with a new you

After cancer, nothing is ever really the same again. Even if you are not troubled with long-term physical side effects as a result of treatment and even if your cancer never comes back, you'll likely find that you are different emotionally and that your standard mode of operating in the world has changed. Read all about that fact in Chapter 20, where we endeavor to help you define yourself anew after cancer.

This is the time that you get to decide all over again who to be, what to say about yourself, and how to make changes in your life that reflect your new perspective on the gift of time. Here, too, are tips on how to protect yourself as you head boldly into your brave new world.

Chapter 2

The Mutants Take Over: A Primer on Cancer

*C*ancer is a loaded word if ever there was one — a word incapable of tip-toeing into a conversation. Instead, the word *cancer* storms in, attracting attention much like an oversized neon sign, every letter blinking in brightest red. No doubt about it, *cancer* is a word that, when spoken aloud, most often overrides just about any other topic.

The word sounds even more urgent if the cancer is yours. When confronted on a personal basis, cancer most often evokes fear. That fear is completely normal. But understand that cancer is not some vicious, drooling alien life form or an enraged, badly dressed ogre in seven-league boots tromping through the countryside of your life.

Cancer is a disease — more accurately, a group of diseases — and every person's body carries within it the possibility of developing cancer.

Cancer also is a disease on the run. Due to the development of more sophisticated detection methods and improved courses of treatment, the number of people surviving cancer in the United States has more than tripled over the past 30 years — so says the National Cancer Institute and the Centers for Disease Control and Prevention (see Figure 2-1).

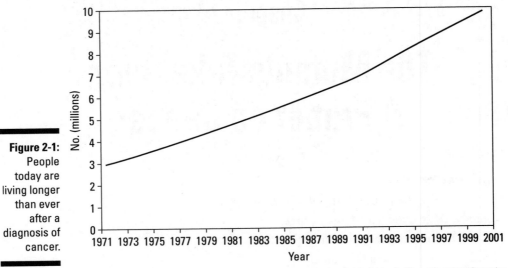

Source: National Cancer Institute and the Centers for Disease Control and Prevention

Figure 2-1: People today are living longer than ever after a diagnosis of cancer.

You can say so, too — it will make you feel better.

In this chapter, you find out what cancer is, what it isn't, and how chemotherapy and radiation work to defeat cancer.

Demystifying the "C" Word

The origin of the word *cancer* is as comical as the connotation is scary.

Studying cancers of the breast, uterus, stomach, and skin in the fifth century, Hippocrates observed that a cancerous tumor (see Figure 2-2) has a hard center with "claw-like projections" — a shape similar to a common crustacean. The good doctor named the disease *karkinos* or *karkinoma,* the Greek word for crab, giving us *carcinoma.* The Latin version of the Greek word is *cancer.*

No wonder cancer makes people crabby!

Hippocrates is, of course, the same Greek physician who gave his name to that famous oath that physicians take upon graduation from medical school.

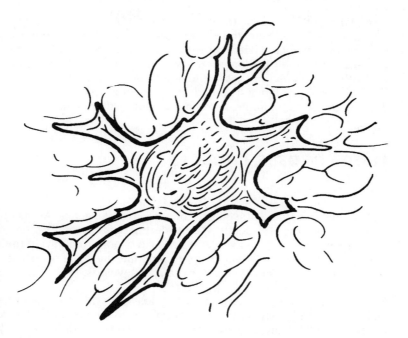

Figure 2-2:
A cancer
cell models
its "claw-
like"
projections.

Understanding how cancer develops

Just what is cancer?

The disease originates at the cellular level. Cells, you may recall from biology class, grow and divide to make sure that you have all the cells you need when you need them to maintain a healthy body. As you read this, some 10 million of your cells are busy dividing. This is normal.

Usually, cell division is an orderly process, with cells growing, maturing, and then dying off as new cells take their place. Sometimes, for reasons not entirely understood, this routine is interrupted. A single cell that has undergone a mutation — either a spontaneous change as a result of a natural incident or one resulting from exposure to a *carcinogen,* or cancer-causing agent — begins to reproduce and keeps at it, without stopping. These new cells, which never reach maturity, form a growth or mass of tissue, and that mass is called a *tumor.*

Tumors come in two types: *benign* (noncancerous) and *malignant:*

 ✔ Generally, benign tumors stay put and do not spread to other parts of the body. If a benign tumor is surgically removed, it usually does not come back.

> ✔ Malignant tumors, on the other hand, contain abnormal cells that continue to divide. Sometimes these cells invade tissue or organs nearby and try to destroy the healthy cells. Sometimes cancerous cells enter the bloodstream or the lymphatic system. When that happens, the cancer cells can spread to sites in the body distant from the site at which the cancer originated. If it spreads, the cancer is termed *metastatic* — more about this topic in the upcoming section "Differentiating among tumors."

What causes cancer?

If only we knew!

Well, actually we know the culprit for some people: genes. As we discuss later in this chapter (see the section "Considering Risk Factors"), about 10 percent of the people who get cancer get it because of abnormalities in their genes. Lots of research is underway to try to pinpoint these abnormalities and find ways to deal with them even before cancer develops.

But unless late-breaking news (reported just after this book went to press) has revealed precisely what it is in our genes that causes cell division to go out of control, for the majority of cancers, no one yet knows exactly why the switch gets stuck when a particular cell turns "on."

Over time, plenty of factors have taken the blame. Some of them, considered identified risk factors, include smoking, an unhealthy diet, and unprotected exposure to the sun's rays. We talk more about these factors later in this chapter. Electromagnetic fields (think cellphones) also have taken the rap, but to date, no conclusive scientific evidence supports the claim. Some rumors about things that cause cancer, such as tight underwired bras and antiperspirants, are just funny. These rumors have no basis in fact, much like the old myths that claimed illness was caused by the brisk night air or excessive personal hygiene.

No one would dispute that having cancer causes stress, but to date there is no evidence that stress is directly responsible for causing cancer. The National Cancer Institute reports that scientists do know that "many types of stress activate the body's endocrine (hormone) system, which in turn can cause changes in the immune system, the body's defense against infection and disease (including cancer)." However, there is no scientific proof that stress-induced changes in the immune system directly cause cancer.

In seeking a place to lay blame for cancer, some people have come to believe that the tragic loss of a spouse or loved one may cause the disease. Not so, says the National Cancer Institute: "Most cancers have been developing for many years and are diagnosed only after they have been growing in the body for a long time (from 2 to 30 years). This fact argues against an association between the death of a loved one and the triggering of cancer." Again, the

Institute reports that "although studies have shown that stress factors alter the way the immune system functions, they have not provided scientific evidence of a direct cause-and-effect relationship between these immune system changes and the development of cancer."

Research, of course, continues.

Listing the types of cancer

Doctors do know that cancer actually is many different diseases, each one complex in its own way. Here, with a nod to the order preferred by the Abramson Cancer Center at the University of Pennsylvania, is a list of some of the different types of cancer. Keep in mind that each type of cancer also has subtypes.

- Bone cancers
- Brain tumors
- Breast cancers
- Endocrine system cancers
- Gastrointestinal cancers
- Gynecologic cancers
- Head and neck cancers
- Leukemia
- Lung cancers
- Lymphomas
- Multiple myeloma
- Pediatric cancers
- Penile cancer
- Prostate cancer
- Sarcomas
- Skin cancers
- Testicular cancer
- Thyroid cancer
- Urinary tract cancers

Here's something else that doctors know for certain: Cancer is not contagious. You didn't "catch" it from anyone else, and your family and friends can't get it from you.

Differentiating among tumors

The types of cancer listed in the previous section are named for common sites where various cancers originate. Many of these cancers may spread to other sites — they may *metastasize* or disseminate to other organs. For example, a breast cancer may spread to the lungs, bones, or brain.

If several organs are affected by cancer when you are diagnosed, a *pathologist* — a doctor who studies tissues with a microscope and who stains those tissues to identify various cellular characteristics — will need to establish the site of the cancer's origin. If you are diagnosed with lung cancer that has metastasized to the adrenal glands, you won't hear the doctors say you have cancer of the adrenal glands. They will say you have lung cancer that has spread, because cancer is always defined according to the primary tumor.

When a cancer has spread, usually the outcome is not as favorable, and treatment may change as well. With few exceptions, the focus of treatment for metastasized cancer is more *systemic,* involving the whole body. Although there are important exceptions, local treatments, such as surgery or radiation, generally are used for relief of symptoms.

If cancer comes back (which you can read about in Chapter 19), it usually is not a new cancer; it contains the same cells found in the original tumor, even if the disease now is in a different part of the body.

Watching the Immune System in Action

Okay — so far, we've said that we know how you *didn't* get cancer, and we've admitted that we don't understand exactly how you *did.* We know a little more about how cancer attacks the body and how the body fights back.

Marvel that it is, the body is programmed to fight infection and disease. Scientists think that the body fights cancer the same way it tries to protect you from viruses. How the immune system works is complicated — there are a lot of characters to keep straight. We promise we won't test you, so read on just for your own enlightenment.

The good guys don't always wear white hats, but your white blood cells are often heroes.

Here's an action-packed scenario of how your immune system works (see Figure 2-3):

1. **When a white blood cell known as a *macrophage* finds a virus, the macrophage devours and digests the virus.**

2. **Flaunting its victory, the macrophage displays bits of the virus on its surface.** These shreds of virus are known as *antigens*.

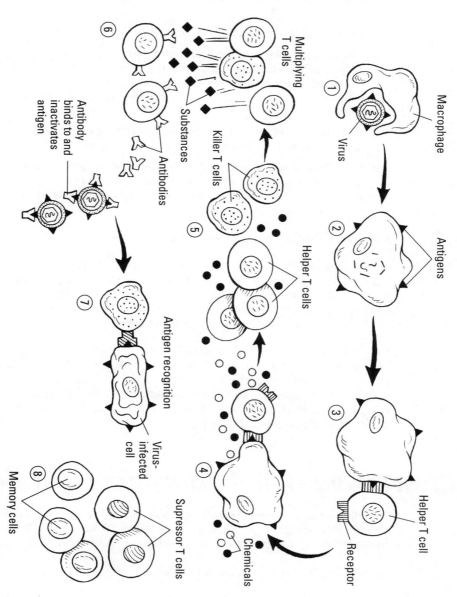

Figure 2-3:
The immune system in action. Imagine all this going on without any conscious assistance!

3. **A particular "helper" T cell, which is another type of white blood cell, notices the antigens on the surface of the macrophage and attaches itself.**

4. **Working together, the macrophage and the T cell produce several chemical substances that result in intercellular communication.**

5. **One of these substances sends signals to other helper T cells and also calls for help from "killer" T cells.** Both types of cells begin to multiply.

6. **The multiplying T cells release substances that cause additional helper cells to multiply and also to produce antibodies that bind to antigens.** These antibodies make it easier for macrophages to destroy viruses. They also signal blood components, called *complement,* to further damage the viruses.

7. **The killer T cells scout around for additional cells in the area that have come under attack by viruses, and they repeat their good works.**

8. **When the immune system determines that the infection is under control, "suppressor" T cells move in and turn off the other cells.** Sentries, in the form of memory cells, stay on duty just in case the same virus mounts another attack.

Sounds something like an adventure movie, doesn't it?

As you may expect, the immune system goes after early cancer cells and destroys them whenever possible. Sometimes, that's not possible — for instance, when there are overwhelming numbers of cancer cells or the cells have mutated in such a way that the immune system does not detect them, which allows the cells to evade immune surveillance.

In a situation where rapidly dividing cancer cells are at work in a body with an impaired immune system, the outlook can be grim. That said, doctors already have some weapons that help to boost an ailing immune system or enable the immune system to focus attention specifically on the cancerous cells. Eventually, they hope to develop even more weapons that will lend additional reinforcement to the troops already on duty.

Discovering How Treatments Fight Back

We talk a lot about *fighting* cancer, because cancer routinely is portrayed as an enemy (and rightly so, because it can kill you). Most of the language used to describe how cancer treatments work is harsh and uses military imagery.

So be it. Let the bugles sound the call to action!

Currently, doctors use four different kinds of treatments to fight cancer. These treatments are

✔ **Surgery:** Surgery, of course, is used to remove a tumor and any tissue around the tumor that may hold cancerous cells. Sometimes, surgery is all the treatment you need.

✔ **Chemotherapy:** Also known as *anticancer drugs,* chemotherapy kills cancer cells (see Figure 2-4). When they're dead, these cells can no longer grow or multiply. The body eliminates the dead cells naturally.

Some chemotherapy is administered before surgery to shrink a tumor. Sometimes, the tumor is removed surgically, and chemotherapy is then used to kill any cancer cells that may have spread elsewhere in the body. Some chemotherapy helps relieve symptoms of cancer, so that patients may live without pain. See Part III of this book for much more information about chemotherapy.

✔ **Radiation therapy:** Radiation therapy stops cancer cells from reproducing. A radiated cell is fried, stopped in its tracks — dead. Again, the body eliminates the dead cells naturally. See Part IV of this book for detailed information about radiation therapy.

In some cases, doctors use only chemotherapy to fight cancer. In other instances, doctors prescribe radiation therapy, either alone or in addition to chemotherapy.

✔ **Biological therapy:** One type of biological therapy helps your immune system destroy cancer cells. Specific drugs are used for specific types of cancers. The drugs you may have heard of include interleukin, interferon, trastuzumab (Herceptin), rituximab (Rituxan), gefitinib (Iressa), erlotonib (Tarceva), and imatinib (Gleevec).

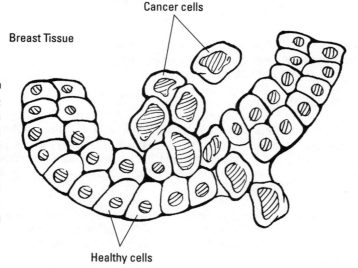

Figure 2-4:
Cancer cells differ in appearance considerably from healthy cells.

Cancer cells

Breast Tissue

Healthy cells

A second kind of biological therapy helps control side effects from other cancer treatments. For example, drugs are available that increase your white blood cell count during chemotherapy, make red blood cells if you have anemia, or manufacture platelets. These drugs fall into a general class of medicines called *growth factors* or *colony stimulating factors*. See Chapter 9 for more information on biological therapy.

Considering Risk Factors

As we mention in the section "What causes cancer?" earlier in the chapter, we know that for some people genes are the culprits. Right now, doctors know that only about 10 percent of all cancers are genetic, or inherited. If you are in that 10 percent — well, you can run, but you can't hide.

What factors contribute to cancer in the other 90 percent of the population? There's no clear-cut answer, but in this section we discuss several well-known factors that may increase the risk of cancer.

Blaming your genes

As scientists begin to understand the human genome more thoroughly, they are slowly but steadily recognizing the genetic mutations that result in cancers. Research is underway right now to try to identify the precise locations of gene abnormalities that lead to cancers. When the locations are mapped, the goal will become to find ways to target these abnormalities with treatments that won't harm other organs.

The more predictable gene abnormalities that scientists detect, the more effective genetic screening becomes, so people at risk for cancer can be identified and treated before cancer develops.

Sounds ideal, doesn't it?

For example, mutations of two genes (known as *BRCA-1* and *BRCA-2*) have been connected to the development of breast and ovarian cancer. There are families with strong histories of pancreatic cancer, malignant melanoma, colorectal, and other cancers. These families have mutations in other specific genes.

If you or your family members have a significant family history of any type of cancer, you want to speak with your doctor about genetic screening, which also can determine other known genetic abnormalities associated with inherited syndromes.

Looking for other causes

Chances are that you're reading this book because you've already been diagnosed with cancer and are preparing for chemotherapy and/or radiation treatments. If so, you need to know that you are *not* to blame.

Maybe you smoke. Maybe you have lung cancer. Maybe you're beating yourself up because you've known for years that scientists have proven a correlation between smoking and lung cancer. But not everyone with a risk factor like smoking (or even with several risk factors) actually gets cancer. In fact, many people who have identified risk factors never develop cancer. Conversely, some people who have no known risk factors at all do develop cancer.

Could you have reduced your risk of cancer by not smoking? Probably. Could you have guaranteed yourself a life without the threat of cancer by not smoking? No.

The only explanation that makes sense is that some complex series of circumstances came into play at the cellular level that caused you to develop cancer. Rather than waste energy blaming yourself for getting cancer, use that energy to help yourself get better.

As you get better, you may develop an interest in living a healthier life. For that reason, we are including here some of the common risk factors for cancer. Think of them as reminders for you to consider after you have completed treatments, or to pass on to family members and friends.

- **Tobacco:** The National Cancer Institute reports that a third of all cancer deaths each year are due to "smoking tobacco, using smokeless tobacco and being regularly exposed to environmental tobacco smoke." Though smokers are at the highest risk for lung cancer, they also are at higher risk for developing other kinds of cancer. The good news is that soon after a smoker quits, the risk of developing cancer begins to drop.

- **Alcohol:** The National Institute on Alcohol Abuse and Alcoholism estimates that 2 to 4 percent of all cancer cases are thought to be caused by excessive consumption of alcohol. What's "excessive"? That depends on many factors — gender, body weight, and family history among them. You probably know better than anyone else when your drinking is out of control.

As time goes by

The first study reporting a connection between smoking and cancer was published in 1950. However, astute physicians practicing in the late 1700s noted an increase in polyps among snuff users and pipe smokers.

✔ **Diet and exercise:** The American Institute for Cancer Research reports that eating a diet high in vegetables, fruits, whole grains, and beans; maintaining a healthy weight; exercising regularly; and not smoking has "a direct and measurable effect on cancer risk." Its report is based on a 13-year study of nearly 30,000 women conducted by the Iowa Women's Health Study and analyzed by researchers at the Mayo Clinic Cancer Center. The report reaped dozens of findings in many areas of women's health. For a look at some of the results, do an Internet search for "Iowa Women's Health Study" and your particular area of interest.

✔ **Ultraviolet (UV) radiation:** The Skin Cancer Foundation has declared that skin cancer has reached epidemic proportions. In the past ten years, the number of cases of *melanoma* — the most serious form of skin cancer — has grown more than any other form of cancer. The Foundation's first rule of protection is this: "Do not sunbathe." If you must go out, the Foundation recommends avoiding "unnecessary sun exposure" between 10 a.m. and 4 p.m., which are "the peak hours for harmful ultraviolet radiation."

✔ **Chemicals:** *The New England Journal of Medicine* published a report in 2000 by researchers who concluded that "environmental exposures far outweigh the role of heredity in causing cancer." Today, most scientists agree that exposure to some pesticides, metals, and chemicals — such as polychlorinated biphenyls and other mixtures of toxic chemicals — may increase the risk of cancer. That also holds true for additives, and for the natural chemicals found in some foods. (That said, some natural chemicals found in fruits and vegetables work in the body to fight cancer.)

✔ **X-ray procedures and medical radiation:** The medical journal *The Lancet,* in January 2004, reported that about 700 of the 124,000 cases of cancer diagnosed each year in the United Kingdom "could be attributable to exposure to diagnostic X-rays," which are said to provide "the largest man-made source of radiation exposure to the general population." Radiation therapy treatments, which can damage healthy cells, also carry a slight risk — but, generally, the benefits of treatment are thought to outweigh the risks. If you are considering going through radiation therapy, your radiation oncologist can help you quantify what the risks of damage to healthy cells may be in your case.

✔ **Hormone replacement therapy (HRT):** For years, doctors routinely prescribed HRT for menopausal women. That changed only recently. In July 2002, *The Journal of the American Medical Association* published the results of a study on conjugated estrogens plus progestins (a type of hormone replacement therapy) that was halted by the National Institutes of Health after safety monitors realized that the participants receiving the drug "had more incidents of breast cancer" and other life-threatening diseases "than those receiving the placebo." (See the sidebar "Women at risk.") Still, some forms of short-term hormone replacement therapy may be helpful for some women suffering from extreme symptoms of menopause. If you are experiencing extreme symptoms, by all means speak with your doctor.

Women at risk

Writing in *The Greatest Experiment Ever Performed on Women: Exploding the Estrogen Myth* (Hyperion), renowned science journalist Barbara Seaman reports that in 1938, a British biochemist published — rather than sold — his formula for oral estrogen in an effort to stop Nazi Germany from cornering the market on synthetic sex hormones. The British biochemist knew that his drug carried a serious risk for endometrial cancer and breast cancer, and he said so.

No one listened.

"Medical policy on estrogens has been to 'shoot first and apologize later' — to prescribe the drugs for a certain health problem and then see if there is a positive result," Seaman writes in her introduction. "Over the years, hundreds of millions, possibly billions of women, from every corner of the world have been lab animals in this unofficial trial. They were not volunteers. They were given no consent forms. And they were put at serious, often devastating, risk."

Controversy — sometimes the raging variety — has circled all around almost every risk factor listed here. One study shows *this* to be true, the next study shows *that*. Remember when you were told that eating a diet high in fiber helped decrease the risk of colon cancer? Now scientists are saying that's not so.

When all is said and done regarding risk factors, it makes sense to want to improve your odds, to be aware of legitimate dangers to your health. Medical science has proven that changes in some personal behaviors can decrease the risk of cancer. However, you don't want to confuse decreasing the risk of developing cancer with actually preventing cancer.

No one can promise that decreasing the *risk* of cancer actually prevents cancer. What it comes down to is cutting your own deal with the risk factors. You decide what risks to take, keeping in mind that these behaviors increase the possibility — but do not guarantee — that cancer will develop.

Looking to the Future: Ongoing Research

Key weapons in the fight against cancer are research and the development of new treatments based on new discoveries. In this section, we identify two areas that are currently of particular interest to scientists.

Targeting genetic culprits

As we mention earlier in the chapter, research continues into the genes and gene products that have been identified as causes of cancer in some people. For example, as we mention in the section "Blaming your genes," scientists know that two genes — *BRCA-1* and *BRCA-2* — are connected to the development of breast and ovarian cancers. Also, a gene known as *HER2/neu,* which helps regulate cell growth, may, if altered, cause particularly aggressive tumor cells. Genes that lead to the growth of blood vessels are also a research target, because blood vessels play a critical role in the *metastatic process* — the process by which cancer spreads from one organ to another.

Cancers caused by genes and gene products may not readily respond to standard chemotherapy treatments, but in some instances new drugs are available, and others are in development. For instance, in clinical trials the drug Herceptin (trastuzumab) has been shown to slow the growth of cancerous tumors in some women who test positive for abnormalities in the HER2/neu gene.

Many doctors believe that the future of oncology lies in identifying additional genetic changes that result in cancer and in developing new drugs aimed at those genes.

Developing fortified antibodies

Another important and growing focus of research aims at identifying tumor *antigens* that are characteristic of various malignant cells. After identifying these tumor antigens (which are like the shreds of virus mentioned in the earlier section "Watching the Immune System in Action"), the goal is to develop fortified antibodies to fight them. This follows the basic principle of treating an infection with antibiotics.

This targeted therapy would use multiple vectors armed with radioactive materials, antibiotics, or chemotherapy drugs to deliver a death blow to the cancer cells. A conjugated compound injected into the bloodstream would target a specific cancer cell type, wherever it may be in the body.

In principle, this type of therapy should work, but the catch is in identifying the antigen, fabricating an antibody, and conjugating it with a radioactive material or chemo agent that won't damage any other cells in the body. The principle is simple, but the execution is complex.

Speaking of the "C" Word

Naming cancer, speaking the six-letter, lowercase word aloud, removes some of its power to terrify. This is better understood today, but up until the mid-1950s, many people chose to whisper the word or to superstitiously refer to it only as "The Big C." Now, the baby boomers, who have proven repeatedly that we will talk about anything, are much more open to discussing cancer.

Psychologically, that's a good approach. Annette L. Stanton, a faculty member at the Jonsson Cancer Center at the University of California at Los Angeles, conducted a study, while in the Department of Psychology at the University of Kansas, on women with breast cancer that shows expressing emotions helped them confront the disease and feel more positive about their health. The study was reported in October 2000 in the *Journal of Consulting and Clinical Psychology*.

Stanton concluded that the 92 women who participated

- ✔ Had fewer medical appointments for cancer-related morbidities
- ✔ Enjoyed enhanced physical health and vigor
- ✔ Showed decreased distress during the next three months compared with those "low in emotional expression"

Stanton's study noted that "expressive coping also was related to improved quality of life for those who perceived their social contexts as highly receptive."

Here's the bottom line: If you don't talk about your cancer, your family and friends will not have the opportunity to be "highly receptive" to your emotional struggles, leaving you to struggle alone.

Practicing saying the word

The word *cancer* may not come easily at first. As in all matters, practice makes perfect. You can go so far as to stand in front of a mirror and repeat the words "I have cancer" until you are more comfortable. When the phrase comes naturally, you can turn your attention to what you plan to do about having cancer. One good answer is this: "Tell the people who care about me."

You do not have to tell everyone you know everything you know. In fact, you may want to work up three or four versions of your "I have cancer" story.

One may be just a few sentences long, short and sweet. Another may consist of several paragraphs of pertinent information. And for some close friends, only the entire story will suffice — if you're in the mood at the moment they ask. You can always offer a short version for now and promise the unexpurgated version at a later date.

You may also choose to tell people who don't know anything about you at all, by taking part in a support group. For help finding such a group, speak with your doctors or see Chapter 17.

Scheduling pity parties

Woe is me! I've got cancer!

Taking time to feel sorry for yourself about your diagnosis is another legitimate way to confront the disease. Spending some time bemoaning this turn of events, this interruption in your life, is perfectly normal. One way to keep from dwelling on the subject day in and day out is to schedule a pity party for yourself from time to time.

At the party — usually the guest list is best limited to just yourself and a spouse or close friend — you give yourself permission to wallow in despair. Shout or curse, punch pillows, or even throw a cheap china figurine (one you never really liked) at a wall. Dissolve into tears and fully experience feeling sorry for yourself. A good time limit for these affairs is about 20 minutes, scheduled throughout the week as needed.

If your emotional state reaches the point where you or a family member suspects serious depression, you may want to consider seeking the help of a psychologist. See Chapter 14 for some guidance on when this step may be necessary.

Tell one, tell all

One woman we know, shortly after receiving her diagnosis, methodically went through her address book and called everyone in it to say she had cancer. A close friend observing this exercise asked why that was necessary.

"If I tell everybody I know, they can all help me in some way," said the woman, still dialing. "I do not intend to go through this alone."

Pity parties, no matter how often you hold them, are not meant to take the place of meaningful discussion about concerns regarding your illness, your treatments, or your specific needs. Pity parties are meant to serve as an occasional outlet for dammed-up frustration.

Though such get-togethers may provide some momentary emotional support, the level of emotional support available to you — and likely required by you — is much higher. You'll get that higher level of support after you've taught yourself to be comfortable talking about your cancer, so name it and claim it.

Comforting the people around you

Unfortunately, just because you become comfortable talking about your cancer doesn't mean that everyone will be comfortable listening. In some instances, you may even be asked to help a person you sought out for emotional support. In other instances, silence may indeed turn out to be golden.

What?

Here I am, the one with cancer, and I should be expected to put other people's feelings before my own?

Well, yes. This is one of the many opportunities you will have while coping with cancer to learn that life goes on, seemingly unconcerned that you're just starting radiation treatments or are wrestling with side effects from chemotherapy.

Some people who love you and want the best for you likely are unaware of the encouraging statistics on survival rates. Upon hearing your news, these people may become profoundly upset and actually turn to you for help.

You have several options. You can help by acknowledging that you know you have upset your friend by saying, "Yes, I know it's upsetting. I'm upset too. I hope you will help me get through this." Doing this brings the discussion back to you. If someone appears inconsolable, you may have to gently point out that you're going through a lot yourself, and encourage your friend to seek solace elsewhere.

Surprisingly, in this day and age, news of your diagnosis may still scare some people. When you tell them, or when they hear the news from someone else, they won't know what to say or what to do. Some of them, even people you may know well, will choose to say and do nothing. A little empathy is required here. Maybe, unknown to you, these people have long harbored a secret fear of cancer or had a bad experience with another friend or relative who had the disease.

You don't have to know why some people can't handle your cancer. You may simply want to note that person's absence from your support team and try not to judge. Months from now, even years from now, these same friends may return to the fold to help you celebrate surviving.

Playing the blame game

As you rejoice in the company of people who do want to help you, you may enjoy playing a perverse and yet satisfying little game. As we've said before, after a diagnosis of cancer, much of life goes on. That means you still will be subject to unexpected joys and unanticipated troubles, all of which have nothing at all to do with your cancer.

Before cancer, coping with a furnace that goes out, a sewer that's backed up, or a washing machine that has decided to skip the spin cycle all are extremely frustrating. After cancer, these and similar events seem downright insulting. As you sit in the car on the side of the highway with the radiator boiling over, you will think to yourself, "Isn't it enough that I have cancer and all my plans for the future are in turmoil?"

Apparently, it isn't enough.

You may well sit on the side of the highway. You may have to clean up a flooded basement, or at least find someone who will do it for you. You may encounter the mother of all paper jams in your printer the morning your report is due. The screen in your third-story window may fall out as you try to wipe away an unsightly spider web.

Frankly, the list of frustrating (and occasionally expensive) events that may occur is endless — events that will demand your attention when your only wish is to lie down on the couch and rest.

Here's the game: Blame it all on cancer. That won't make any of the problems go away, but you can use your anger or irritation about them to help fuel any anger or irritation you may have about cancer. So often, despair leads only to an accelerated schedule of pity parties, whereas anger sometimes can be transformed into energy to help you cope with cancer.

Play the blame game, and move toward winning.

Keeping Your Sense of Humor

Don't forget to pack your sense of humor on your journey through cancer treatments. Humor can be a powerful weapon. Whether you are comfortable with the military metaphors or you prefer a more peaceful theme, humor will serve you well as you, your doctors, and your treatments work to destroy your cancer.

Lila Green, a self-described "humor educator" and a survivor of ovarian cancer, says that humor "helps give perspective — it gives distance." Speaking to the faculty and staff of the Comprehensive Cancer Center at the University of Michigan, Green compared humor to changing a baby's diaper. "It doesn't solve the problem," she said, "but it sure makes things better for the moment."

John Whelpley would agree. Another cancer survivor, Whelpley operates a Web site called Tumor Humor (`www.whelpley.com/tumor_humor.htm`), where he offers cancer-related jokes and discusses the many physiological benefits of laughter. A good belly laugh — or even an earnest fit of the giggles — can do the following:

- Reduce stress
- Stimulate your circulatory system
- Stimulate your immune system
- Increase your heart rate
- Boost your breathing
- Provide temporary pain relief
- Promote well-being

Laughing through the centuries

Historical documents show that surgeons even as far back as the 13th century tried using humor to distract patients from the pain of surgery. (Those must have been some hilarious jokes!) The American Cancer Society reports that "Humor was also widely used and studied by the medical community in the early 20th century."

The Society also relates the story of the late Norman Cousins, longtime editor of the *Saturday Review.* The ailing Cousins checked himself out of a hospital and into a hotel, where he watched funny movies and read funny books, laughing his way back to health.

The American Cancer Society considers humor "a complementary tool to promote health and cope with illness." The Society also reports that many hospitals and ambulatory care centers have special rooms "where humorous materials, and sometimes people, are there to help make people laugh." Among the commonly used materials are movies, audio and videotapes, books, games, and puzzles.

Hey, it can't hurt!

Chapter 3

You Will Be Tested: What All Those Tests Show

As you prepare for your journey through cancer treatments, more than once you may stop along the road and ask yourself, "Is it true? Do I really have cancer? Is there a chance that the doctor is wrong?"

This response is natural, especially if you happen to feel good and have no visible indication that cancer is in your body. Still, almost inevitably, the answer is that the doctor is not wrong and you do have cancer. That's because doctors don't guess when it comes to cancer. They do tests, and then they do more tests to confirm and expand on the information revealed by the first tests.

Maybe an unexpected discovery during a routine physical exam led to your diagnosis. Maybe you developed one or more symptoms that made you or your doctor suspect cancer. Or maybe your cancer was discovered during a recommended screening test. In any case, when doctors suspect cancer, they turn into detectives and follow the clues until they have specific answers.

What happens after the doctor reaches a conclusion and delivers a diagnosis? The answer shouldn't come as a surprise — more tests!

After you've been diagnosed with cancer, tests can provide important information that determines what sort of treatment will work best for you. So roll up your sleeve for that blood test, schedule that biopsy, and make that appointment for an imaging scan. No cheating allowed! You want the best information available from these tests so that you and your detective — er, doctor — can make the best treatment plan possible.

In this chapter, you find out about the kinds of tests that you likely will undergo.

Passing a Battery of Tests

In school, maybe your forte was multiple-choice quizzes. Or maybe you preferred essay tests. One thing is for sure — you were always relieved when the test was open book! Tests designed to provide information about your cancer are not, thank goodness, based on any body of knowledge that you may or may not have retained since your school days, so you can relax on that count.

Mainly, the tests that your doctor schedules for you to help determine the status of your cancer require only your presence.

Having blood drawn

You most certainly will be sent to a laboratory for blood tests, both before chemotherapy and radiation begin and throughout treatment.

 If you are worried that your veins will neglect to pop up and make themselves easily available to the technician, try playing a little air guitar in the parking lot before you go in the building, or even in the hall before you go in the laboratory. Pick the arm the technician most likely will stick and swing it in full circles, backwards and forwards, to make sure the blood is flowing freely. Is this a guarantee that the stick will be easier? Of course not, but it can't hurt.

If needles make you nervous, this may be a good time to talk yourself out of that. Not out of the tests themselves — for there will be many blood tests — but out of being nervous.

Some people are nervous about needles because they associate them with pain. Depending on your past experiences, you may think that having blood drawn is no big deal, or you may think it's terribly painful. Sometimes, putting an experience in perspective can help you think differently about it. Compared to having a baby without drugs, slamming your hand in the closet door, or having a broken bone reset, having blood drawn isn't so terrible. Maybe you can consider it comparable to that momentary discomfort that you feel when you accidentally hit your "funny bone." The sensation is strong at first and then ebbs.

Another suggestion is to listen carefully when the technician says, "Now there will be a little stick" — and choose to believe it.

No one ever said that you have to watch the technician draw your blood. Look at the ceiling, look at the opposite wall, look back over your shoulder at a colorful calendar. To avoid feeling queasy, look anywhere but at your arm or hand. This isn't a test about how tough you are, so if you are more comfortable looking elsewhere, do so.

Some blood tests show your blood count or the general function of some organs. Other blood tests measure substances, called *tumor markers,* that can indicate the presence of specific types of cancer and can indicate whether your treatments are having the desired effect.

Here are some common tumor markers:

- Carcinoembryonic antigen
- Carbohydrate antigen 125, 19-9, 27-29, or 15-3
- Prostate-specific antigen
- Human chorionic gonadotropin
- Alpha-fetoprotein
- 5-hydroxy indole acetic acid
- Serum paraproteins

Stretching out on a table

High-tech pictures provide invaluable information about the size, shape, and location of a tumor. Several different kinds of imaging scans may aid your doctor in planning the best treatment for you.

For some scans, you may be injected with a small amount of radioactive material to better highlight the tissue or organs being scanned. If that's the case, your doctor will tell you about any short-term restrictions you must follow until the material leaves your body.

Some of the tests take time, and others can be completed fairly quickly — it all depends on the type and purpose of the scan, the age of the equipment used, and whether the technician sees something that requires a second look. After the scan, you may be asked to stick around long enough so the technician and the doctor can be certain they have all the images they need.

Imaging scans don't hurt, though lying still on a hard table can become uncomfortable if the scan takes a while.

Some of the imaging machines are noisy, making whirring or clicking noises throughout the scan. You may be offered a choice of radio stations to be piped in through speakers near your head, but often the sounds of the machine will prevent you from concentrating on anything else.

Here are the basics about five different imaging techniques:

✔ **Computer-assisted tomography scan:** Better known as a CT or CAT (for *computed axial tomography*) scan, this type of test uses a computer linked to an x-ray machine. The scan provides cross-section images of your bones, soft tissue, organs, brain, and blood vessels (see Figure 3-1). These images, or "slices," reveal the size and location of a tumor.

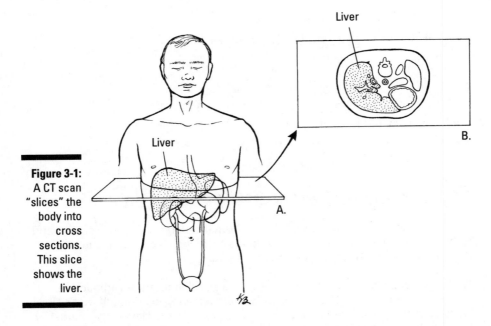

Figure 3-1:
A CT scan "slices" the body into cross sections. This slice shows the liver.

✔ **Positron emission tomography scan:** Also known as a PET scan, this scan may do a better job than a CT scan of finding some (but not all) types of cancer cells and determining what actions those cells are taking. (A machine that does both CT scanning and PET scanning now is available, combining the best of both, but few medical centers have the machine at this time.)

Also, PET scans sometimes are used to help stage cancer, assess response to treatment, or, in the case of a possible recurrence, show the difference between scar tissue and active cancer tissue. PET scans also are useful for planning radiation therapy.

Before the scan, you may be injected with a radioactive tracer, but the amount of radiation is small and will quickly leave your body. Drink a lot of water throughout the day to help your body eliminate it.

✔ **Radionuclide scan:** In some instances, you may be asked to swallow, or have an injection of, a radioactive substance. A scanner measures radioactivity levels in your organs, which allows the doctor to detect abnormal areas based on the amount of radioactivity. Don't worry about the radioactive material remaining in your body after the test. Again, drink a lot of water, and your body will eliminate the material through your urine.

✔ **Ultrasonography:** Ultrasound uses high-frequency sound waves that scan the body and then bounce back to produce an image called a *sonogram*. To produce the images, a technician rubs a chilled gel on your skin and then moves a small imaging wand back and forth over your skin, through the gel. The images appear on a monitor and can be printed to provide specific information for your doctor.

✔ **Magnetic resonance imaging:** Also known as an MRI, magnetic resonance imaging uses a magnet linked to a computer to produce detailed images of the body. These images also can be viewed on a monitor and printed.

Many MRI machines require that you lie inside a narrow metal tube. If you're not claustrophobic, that's not a problem. From time to time, the technician will announce how many minutes more remain to complete the scan. Also, you will be given a buzzer, or panic button, to summon the technician if you become uneasy. If that happens, by all means press the button! You won't be the first person to do so — or the last.

Neglecting to notify the one person who can relieve your anxiety will only add to it. Your rational mind may continue to insist that you are perfectly fine, but if your adrenaline starts pumping and your emotions insist that you are in a "fight or flight" situation, summon the technician and take a minute to calm yourself. No one will think less of you.

Nor does such an interruption mean you have to start all over, as long as you are willing to resume after calming yourself. Normally, if you ask to stop, the technician will tell you just how much time is needed to complete the scan, and you may decide whether to continue. If you choose to leave, you may have to start all over another day.

If the idea of lying in a narrow metal tube while a noisy machine takes pictures of your insides scares you as much as having cancer in the first place, ask your doctor where you might have the test with an MRI machine that has open sides (see Figure 3-2).

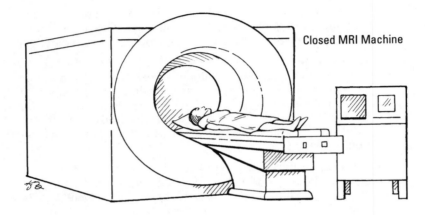

Closed MRI Machine

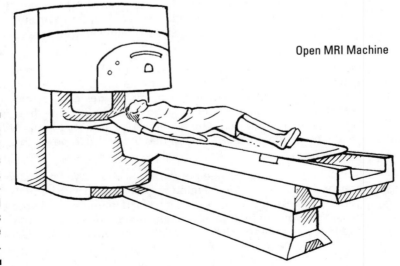

Open MRI Machine

Figure 3-2:
Some MRI machines are tubular, but open-sided MRI machines also are available.

Would you like that sliced?

Computed tomography scans deliver pictures of the body divided into tidy slices or cross sections. Knowing that, it should come as no surprise that the machine takes its name from the Greek words *tomos,* which means "slice," and *graphia,* which means "describing."

Two scientists — Godfrey Hounsfield, a British engineer, and Allan Cormack, a physicist at Tufts University — independently invented the CT scan in 1972. Originally, CT scanners were used only to capture images of the head, but over time the testing method was revised to take pictures of the entire body. Originally, the process took several hours, but today the images are captured in seconds, and the entire test can be over in a matter of minutes.

Undergoing a biopsy

Having tissue removed is practically standard procedure for anyone with cancer. This tissue removal is called a *biopsy,* which is another type of test that provides information about your cancer. For instance, a biopsy reveals the cellular composition of a tumor, and that information may hold clues to the virulence of the tumor.

Biopsies of tumors also provide what is known as a *grade,* or an indication of the degree to which malignant cells resemble healthy cells. In other words, the grade denotes the aggressiveness of the cancer cells. A tumor can be graded from 1 to 3 or 4. Low-grade malignancies tend to be less aggressive; high-grade tumors are more so.

Also, along with other tests, biopsies help your doctor determine the *stage,* or the extent, of your cancer. You can have a very early stage cancer that is high grade, or aggressive. See "Setting the Stage for Treatment," later in this chapter, for more information on staging.

How is the tissue removed during a biopsy? One of three ways, depending on the type of cancer you have:

✔ **Needle biopsy:** A doctor inserts a long, hollow needle at the site of the tumor to remove a small amount of tissue. You may feel pressure, but a local anesthesia prevents you from feeling any pain. Typically, needle biopsies are brief, and they take place in a doctor's office, outpatient surgery suite, or radiology department.

Though you have to be present for a needle biopsy, you do not have to watch. The needle is big, and closing your eyes may make you more comfortable about the experience.

✔ **Surgical biopsy:** If your doctor suspects that you have a cancerous tumor, the surgeon may remove a small part of the tumor for further tests. Surgical biopsies take place at an outpatient surgical center or a hospital. Generally speaking, surgical biopsies require an IV drip and then a trip to the operating room where you likely will receive local anesthesia. You also may be lightly sedated.

✔ **Endoscopy biopsy:** An endoscopy is a test that allows the doctor to examine areas inside the body through a long lighted tube. The equipment allows the doctor to take pictures and, sometimes, to remove suspicious tissue or cells. Endoscopy tests take place at an outpatient surgical center or a hospital, and you will be lightly sedated.

Before a surgical biopsy or endoscopy biopsy, your doctor will tell you how much time to allow for the procedure, and whether you will feel like heading to work or going on about your day afterward. Also, she may prescribe a mild pain reliever for you and/or recommend that you use ice on the incision to keep down any swelling.

What your doctor may not tell you is that frozen peas work better than ice. Before the biopsy, buy a big bag of frozen peas. Divide the peas into individual plastic sandwich bags and throw them back in the freezer. You'll find that a bag of frozen peas more easily takes on the shape of your biopsied body part than any bag of ice. Usually the icing routine is 20 minutes on and 20 minutes off, but check with your doctor about that. You can refreeze your bags of peas over and over.

It's normal to be nervous about any kind of medical test, and it's impossible to ignore that biopsies are most often scheduled to investigate or confirm the presence of cancer. That said, the tests themselves are done under the strictest of controlled circumstances with the highest attention possible paid to safety measures. In other words, it is highly unlikely — repeat, *highly unlikely* — that a biopsy will cause cancer to spread.

Playing the Waiting Game

What is highly likely is that the results of any tests scheduled to determine or confirm whether you have cancer will not be available quickly. This is extremely frustrating, even when you understand why these things take time.

Why *do* these things take time?

Test results from lab work or imaging procedures — yours and everyone else's — have to be checked, double-checked, and analyzed. A report has to be typed up and sent to your doctor. After the report has been received, the doctor has to make time to read it, synthesize the information, and look at other factors in your case or consult additional test results to get the big picture.

Worse, tissues and cells removed during biopsies often need time (we're talking days or even weeks) to be processed and stained with a battery of dyes and other substances in the laboratory before the pathologist can make a conclusive examination. Sometimes, when the diagnosis is not clear-cut, the pathologist may decide to use special stains to help clarify the diagnosis, which may take a week or more. A pathologist may also send your biopsy slides to a more experienced colleague for confirmation, which can delay the process further. Then, as with test results from lab work or imaging scans, the pathologist must check, double-check, and analyze the tissues. Again, a report has to be typed up and sent to your doctor. After the report has been received . . . well, you know the rest.

Maybe your "big picture" is positive and your relationship with your doctor is sufficiently close that he will choose to call you with the test results. Maybe your "big picture" isn't so good, or maybe it's just particularly complex, and your doctor will prefer that you make an appointment to go over all the test results.

The only thing that's certain when it comes to tests and test results is that it will take longer to get the information than you would ever hope.

That said, putting up with the jitters as you wait for correct information still beats the heck out of getting an early report — either good or bad — that tells only part of the story or, worse, tells it wrong. If that happens, you may have to cope with the additional emotional burden of hearing a second set of test results quite different from the first! Keeping that scenario in mind may help you be more patient when waiting for your test results.

Setting the Stage for Treatment

After you've undergone many a test — but before treatments begin — the doctor will want to know the *stage,* or the extent, of your cancer. Staging, a system of assigning a number according to national medical standards, indicates the extent of the cancer and determines the components of your treatment plan.

How do doctors stage your cancer? They take the following factors into consideration:

- ✔ Results from imaging tests
- ✔ Results from biopsies
- ✔ Results from blood tests
- ✔ The location of the tumor
- ✔ Results from your physical examination
- ✔ The grade (aggressiveness) of the cancer

Correct staging is not only important; it's imperative. Generally, there are four stages of cancer, indicated by a number:

- ✔ Stage I indicates a small tumor that has not spread to other organs.

- ✔ Stage II likely means the cancer has not spread, but the tumor is larger or has invaded deeper than a Stage I tumor, or there may be cancer cells in nearby lymph nodes.

- ✔ Stage III indicates that the tumor is even larger, the tumor has a higher grade of cells, and/or some lymph nodes are affected.

- ✔ Stage IV denotes a large tumor that has spread, or *metastasized,* to major organs in the body.

After the staging has been determined, plans can be made for treatment. For instance, if the cancer is small and in one location, sometimes a *local* treatment — surgery or surgery followed by radiation therapy — will be sufficient. If the cancer has spread, the doctor will recommend a *systemic* treatment, such as chemotherapy, which circulates through the body in the bloodstream. (See Chapter 4 for more information on chemotherapy.) If at the time of diagnosis the cancer is Stage IV, you have fewer options. Indeed, you may opt for palliative care, which means that the doctor will provide less aggressive therapies that induce fewer side effects and preserve quality of life. If the prognosis is not good, the doctor may speak to you about hospice care, which we address in detail in Chapter 19.

Sometimes, cancer is staged in such a way that you have the option of either local treatment or systemic treatment. If that happens, you may want to request that another pathology specialist review your case, or you may want to seek out a second opinion to hear another doctor's perspective. (Read more about second opinions in Chapter 4.) The more information you have, the better — especially when you are making such an important decision, which may affect the rest of your life.

Hearing your numbers

Doctors tend to like numbers because they function as a standardized language of sorts. Some people speak that language; others barely know how to say "Hello" or "Another beer, please." When you ask your doctor about your prognosis, the answer may come back in numbers. You are likely to hear your stage, your grade, and the latest statistics for people with the same stage or grade.

If your numbers happen to be really good, the statistics can be comforting. If your numbers are not so good — even middling to so-so — then the statistics can, simply put, drive you crazy.

Here's one way to look at the numbers: A certain number of people win the lottery. A certain number of people get in car accidents on the way to work. A certain number of people give birth to triplets. Maybe you play the lottery. Maybe you drive to work. Maybe you're pregnant, or you were at one time.

So will you be the one who wins, wrecks the car, or has to buy three baby strollers?

Maybe. Maybe not.

Ignoring your numbers

In 2000, there were 9.6 million Americans alive who had experienced cancer. Ask your doctor, and she will tell you that some of these 9.6 million people had numbers that were less than spectacular. As it happens, many factors come into play when a prognosis is calculated. Here are some of them:

- Age
- Stage of cancer
- Response to treatment
- General health
- Performance status (level of activity)
- Unforeseen developments

That last one covers a lot of territory, including strokes of luck (good and bad), the availability of more potent treatments for some types of cancer, and circumstances that some people call miracles. Even if you don't believe in miracles, you do have to believe that statistics don't define you, and numbers don't know you.

Think of it this way: If someone you know who is your same age got the same kind of cancer you have, would you expect your treatments, your experiences, or your recoveries to be exactly the same?

Of course not. Everyone is different, and every case of cancer is different, in ways large and small.

People diagnosed with cancer get no guarantees about how long they will live. But neither do people who have not been diagnosed with cancer! With that revelation in mind, don't let your numbers run — or ruin — your life, especially if you don't like them and they don't like you. No less a hero than Han Solo of *Star Wars* fame would say the same. In *Star Wars* (the original film, which came out in 1977 and is now called *Episode IV*), there is a delicious moment when the droid C-3PO recites the statistical probability of successfully maneuvering through an asteroid field — right at the moment when Solo is trying to do just that. Solo snaps, "Never tell me the odds!"

Good advice, that.

So put your energy into making room in your life for cancer and embracing the treatments designed to make you well. (See Chapter 20 for more on concentrating on what really matters.)

Recognizing Symptoms of Cancer

Many, many people are surprised when they learn they have cancer. Maybe you were one of them. Or, maybe you had one or more symptoms that led you to believe you needed to get to a doctor.

Some of the symptoms of cancer, such as a lump in the breast or unusual bleeding or discharge from assorted body parts, are well known. Some are less well known, but all recognizable symptoms represent a call for help from the body. You do yourself a favor when you report such symptoms to your doctor so he can order the necessary tests.

For future reference — and our wish is that you never again need this information for yourself or your family — here is a list of symptoms that may signal the presence of cancer:

✔ A thickening of tissue in any part of the body

✔ A recognizable change in a wart or mole

✔ A sore that does not heal

✔ A nagging cough or hoarseness

✔ A cough that produces blood

✔ A change in bowel or bladder habits

✔ A difficulty swallowing or frequent indigestion

✔ An unexplained weight loss or gain

✔ A discharge or unusual bleeding

✔ A lingering feeling of fatigue

✔ A high fever that lasts for several weeks

Resisting the urge to self-diagnose

Okay, you've just read over the list and you've started to fret. This symptom sounds familiar, or you've experienced that one. Fear creeps in. The imagination fires up. You begin to self-diagnose. Suddenly, you are certain that you are doomed.

Hold everything!

You're not a doctor, even if you have seen one on television. But you *have* a doctor — a real one, not an actor. Why not present the problem to that person and either have your fears put to rest or get a diagnosis based on fact?

The symptoms on this list may have causes that are in no way related to cancer. But if you experience them for many days or weeks, or longer, they're almost certainly indications of some health problem, and you'd be wise to get them checked out.

Analyzing pain

Some people think that pain is a symptom of cancer. Others think that early cancer does not cause pain. Both schools of thought may be correct, depending on the type of cancer. Some types of cancer that may involve pain include

✔ Bladder cancer

✔ Bone cancer

- ✔ Brain cancer
- ✔ Kidney cancer
- ✔ Leukemia
- ✔ Non-Hodgkin's lymphoma
- ✔ Oral cancer
- ✔ Pancreatic cancer
- ✔ Prostate cancer
- ✔ Stomach cancer
- ✔ Uterine cancer

Again, resist the urge to self-diagnose. If you experience pain over a period of time that strikes you as too long, call your doctor and schedule the tests that can provide answers.

Appreciating Early Detection

If you are one of those people whose cancer was detected early because of a screening test — well, good for you! Part of the reason that the number of cancer survivors in the United States has more than tripled in the last 30 years (and it has) is because of early detection. In general, the sooner that cancer — any kind of cancer — is detected, the sooner your doctors can bring out the big guns and go after it.

Though some people are still averse to "looking for something that may not be there," government and private health agencies, along with doctors, are working hard every day to promote screening tests for different types of cancer. As the educational efforts pay off and people more readily embrace the idea of monitoring the status of their health, more individuals get screened, more cancer is detected earlier, and more people continue to boost the survival statistics. That's all good news.

Of course, after you've been diagnosed with and treated for cancer, you can be sure that your health will be carefully monitored for years to come. Don't be surprised, then, if your doctor recommends regular cancer screening tests for you, in addition to the typical follow-up tests that you will be requested to take over the years (see Chapter 19).

Knowing the types of screening tests

The "gold standard" for cancer screening tests, the benchmark by which such tests are measured, is whether screening leads to a significant reduction in death rates.

For a multitude of reasons — among them cost, reliability, and ease — the medical profession has not developed and promoted screening tests for all types of cancer. Endometrial, ovarian, and oral cancer are among the types of cancer for which no standard screening tests are proven to be beneficial. That's not to say these cancers can't be diagnosed with the help of certain blood tests, biopsies, or x-rays. They can. But doctors rarely order the tests unless they suspect cancer.

Common sense should tell you that if you have a family history of cancer, you should alert your doctor to that fact and proceed as directed.

Here are some of the types of cancer for which you can be screened. Again, screening may be how your cancer was found. If that's the case, just give the pertinent paragraph a nod of appreciation as you read further. On the other hand, you may be asked to schedule one or more of these screening tests in the years to come as a way of monitoring your health after cancer.

- **Breast cancer:** A *mammogram* is an x-ray image that can find tiny tumors too small to be felt during a self-exam or a manual exam by a doctor (see Figure 3-3). The American Cancer Society recommends that women 40 and older have a mammogram once a year. Younger women are advised to have a manual breast examination by a doctor every three years unless the disease runs in the family, in which case, they should speak with a doctor about having mammograms.

- **Cervical cancer:** A *Pap test* is a painless procedure performed by a doctor who scrapes cells from the cervix. The American College of Obstetricians and Gynecologists recommends that young women get their first Pap test within three years after becoming sexually active or by age 21, whichever comes first. Through the age of 30, women should schedule annual Pap tests. After that, women with three consecutive normal tests can wait two or three years before the next Pap test. Of course, women with a history of cervical cancer will want to be screened more often.

- **Colon and rectal cancer:** The most effective screening test is a *colonoscopy,* in which a thin, lighted tube examines the rectum and colon while the patient is under mild sedation. This test is recommended for anyone over 50, whether or not there is a family history of the disease. A less invasive but less thorough test, called a *sigmoidoscopy,* also is available. Blood in the stool, sometimes a symptom of cancer, can be detected by a fecal occult blood test. A barium enema enhances x-rays of the colon and rectum. A digital rectal exam is another means of screening for abnormalities.

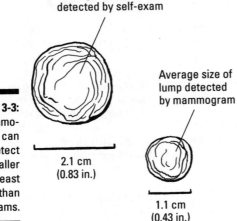

Average size of lump
detected by self-exam

Average size of
lump detected
by mammogram

Figure 3-3:
Mammo-
grams can
detect
smaller
breast
tumors than
self-exams.

2.1 cm
(0.83 in.)

1.1 cm
(0.43 in.)

✔ **Prostate cancer:** A digital rectal exam allows a doctor to feel for changes in the prostate gland. A blood test for prostate-specific antigens (PSA) also can detect a problem. Some controversy has arisen over the value of screening for prostate cancer, but most health professionals and organizations continue to recommend a digital rectal exam and a PSA once a year for all men over 50 and for men over 40 who have a history of cancer in the family.

✔ **Skin cancer:** Most people now know that unprotected exposure to the sun is asking for trouble, but most people also remain seduced by the appeal of a rich tan. The Skin Cancer Foundation is ringing the alarm. In the past ten years, the number of cases of *melanoma* — the most serious form of skin cancer — has grown more than any other form of cancer. For a low-tech screening with a high return, visit a dermatologist (a skin doctor) once a year for a whole-body exam.

Redirecting anger about tests

The need to know motivates a lot of people to get regular cancer screening tests. The need not to know, an emotional point of view sometimes adopted by people who have an uneasy relationship with personal health, can be equally strong.

Maybe you had symptoms and you needed to know why. Maybe no symptoms were present, but you believe in trying to take care of yourself. Either way, you went to your doctor, you were tested, and you were told you have cancer.

Even if originally you believed that knowing was better than not knowing, you may become angry after learning your diagnosis. (See Chapter 14 for more on emotional states of mind during cancer.) Out of nowhere, you may suddenly think, "If I hadn't had the test, I wouldn't be going through all this now, rearranging my entire life to make room for cancer treatments." That thought can make you hot under the collar.

Go ahead. Get hot. Get mad, really mad. Let off steam. Then, put yourself back together emotionally. When you are calm again, remind yourself that the earlier cancer is diagnosed, the easier it is to treat — and be grateful for all those tests.

The man behind the Pap test

More than 50 million women have Pap tests each year, many of them as part of a routine gynecological checkup. Some women are unaware that the test screens for cancer, and few know the history of the test.

In 1923, Dr. George N. Papanicolaou, a native of Greece, discovered that women with uterine cancer exhibited "abnormal cells, with enlarged, deformed, or hyperchromatic nuclei." The doctor, then working as a research biologist at Cornell Medical College, considered the discovery "thrilling," but his colleagues were less enthusiastic, saying that much already was known about uterine cancer diagnosis.

In 1943, Dr. Papanicolaou, along with Dr. Herbert F. Traut, published a study that showed how a vaginal smear could detect lesions "in their incipient, pre-invasive phase." That study, according to the American Society for Clinical Pathology, "was a turning point in management of cervical cancer, the most deadly form of cancer in women at the time." Within 20 years, "cervical cancer went from the first to third most deadly form of cancer."

In 1961, Dr. Papanicolaou was named director of the Papanicolaou Cancer Research Institute in Miami. He died the next year, at the age of 79.

Part II
Your Choices along the Way: Making Good Ones

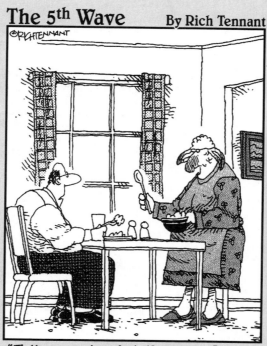

The 5th Wave   By Rich Tennant

"Tell me again what the goal of the clinical trial is?"

In this part . . .

What exactly are chemotherapy and radiation, and how do they work? This part gives you the answers. Also, we fill you in on clinical trials, which set the standard for the future of cancer treatments, and introduce you to the miracle of bone marrow transplants.

Chapter 4

Defining Chemotherapy: The Anticancer Drugs

Chemotherapy, or anticancer drug therapy, is a *systemic* treatment for cancer, which means that chemotherapy drugs move through the blood-stream to all parts of the body.

Time was when the word *chemotherapy* elicited almost as much fear as the word *cancer.* People heard "chemotherapy" and shuddered, because this particular treatment had a reputation for being as hard on the body as cancer itself. In some circles today, chemotherapy still is thought of as poison.

No doubt about it, chemotherapy is strong medicine. It has to be. The job of chemotherapy is to cure or control cancer, a disease that kills 1,500 Americans every day, according to the National Cancer Institute. One big reason more people *don't* die of cancer is the effectiveness of chemotherapy.

There's no question that undergoing chemotherapy can be rough. But many drugs have been developed to help offset some of the more disabling side effects of chemotherapy. Also, for a host of reasons, every individual responds to chemotherapy differently, so "rough" can range from profound fatigue to hospitalization. You may want to decide that instead of fearing chemotherapy, you will simply respect it for its power — and its possibilities.

In this chapter, we introduce you to different chemotherapy regimens and offer some guidelines on working with your doctor to choose the best one for you.

Getting Some Chemotherapy Basics

Chemotherapy, administered under the direction of a medical oncologist with assistance from angels otherwise known as chemo nurses, covers a wide range of drug regimens that all produce side effects. (See Chapters 10 and 11 for a discussion of these side effects.) Most people undergoing chemotherapy do have to alter some aspects of their lives to accommodate the treatments and the side effects, though many people continue to work and carry out most of their family responsibilities. For a number of reasons — chiefly the possibility of an improved outcome — some people even opt to undergo chemotherapy and radiation therapy at the same time, if both are indicated.

We mention in Chapter 2 that cancer routinely is portrayed as an enemy — rightly so, because it can kill you — and most of the language used to describe how cancer treatments work is harsh and makes use of military imagery. Following that metaphor, chemotherapy is a special battalion dispatched to the frontlines, withdrawn, and then dispatched again every couple of weeks until the enemy is at bay.

In civilian language, this means that your chemotherapy treatments are scheduled in cycles, maybe every three or four weeks, with time in between for your body to recover. How many different assaults — er, treatments — will be required depends on several factors. Among them are

- The kind of cancer
- The kind of drugs used
- Your age
- Your general health
- Your body's response to the drugs

That last factor, of course, is monitored by your medical oncologist. If you do well, your series of chemotherapy treatments will take place one after another, following logically from the first to the last. However, if chemotherapy is particularly tough for you, your doctor may spread out the treatments, try a different drug or combination of drugs, or perhaps halt chemotherapy altogether.

Only time will tell.

Sorting out the different drugs

More than 50 different chemotherapy drugs are available to treat cancer. All of them kill cancer cells, though they work in different ways. Generally speaking, all the drugs are designed to go after chemical substances within cancer cells and to interfere with cellular activity during specific phases of the cells' growth cycles. In the process, chemotherapy drugs also kill healthy cells, and that's why side effects develop. Of course, not all drugs work well for all cancers, and in many cases, a combination of chemotherapy drugs is the best course of treatment.

Do you need to know all this information?

Not really. Technically, all you need to know is which chemotherapy drug or combination of drugs your doctor recommends and why. Actually, some people don't want even that much information. Others want to do independent research in order to learn as much as they can about cancer and cancer treatments. You know which kind of person you are, and you should act accordingly.

If you're the type of person who wants the details about the treatment you'll be receiving, we'll get you started. Researchers have divided the available chemotherapy drugs into categories based on how they work. Here are some of the different types of drugs used, the kinds of cancer they are used to treat, and some of the drug names:

- **Antibody-based therapies:** These new agents are aimed at molecular targets. To continue with the military metaphor, these are truly the magic bullets of oncology because they hone in on cancer cells, sparing most normal cells. Currently, antibody-based agents are used to treat breast cancer, colon cancer, lung cancer, lymphoma, and several types of leukemia, but additional targeted therapies are being developed. Ultimately, many other cancers will likely be treated with antibody-based therapies as well. Some of the drugs in use now include trastuzumab, bevacizumab, cetuximab, gefitinib, imatinib, rituximab, and erlotinib.

- **Alkylating agents:** These anticancer drugs act directly on a cell's DNA, which prevents further cell division. Alkylating agents are used against chronic leukemia; non-Hodgkin's lymphoma; Hodgkin's disease; multiple myeloma; and some cancers of the lung, breast, and ovary. Some of the drugs in use are chlorambucil, cyclophosphamide, cisplatin, carboplatin, thiotepa, and busulfan.

- **Nitrosoureas:** These drugs act in a way similar to alkylating agents, interfering with enzymes that help repair DNA. Nitrosoureas are used to treat brain tumors, non-Hodgkin's lymphoma, multiple myeloma, and malignant melanoma. Some of the drugs in use are carmustine and lomustine.

✔ **Antimetabolites:** These drugs alter the function of enzymes required for cell metabolism and protein synthesis, starving the cells to death. Antimetabolites are used in cases of acute and chronic leukemia and tumors of the breast, ovary, and gastrointestinal tract. Some of the drugs in use are 5-fluorouracil, capecitabine, methotrexate, gemcitabine, cytarabine, and fludarabine.

✔ **Antitumor antibiotics:** These drugs bind with DNA and prevent the synthesis of ribonucleic acid (RNA), which is imperative for cell survival. Antitumor antibiotics are used to treat many different cancers. Some of the drugs in use are dactinomycin, daunorubicin, doxorubicin, epirubicin, idarubicin, and mitoxantrone.

✔ **Mitotic inhibitors:** These drugs, derived from plants, halt cell reproduction by inhibiting cell division and prohibiting the use of certain proteins required for mitosis. Mitotic inhibitors are used to treat leukemia, lymphomas, and lung and breast cancers. Some of the drugs in use are paclitaxel, docetaxel, vinblastine, vincristine, and vinorelbine.

In some circumstances, corticosteroids, or natural hormones and hormone-like drugs, also are used to treat such cancers as lymphoma, leukemia, and multiple myeloma. Some of the drugs in use are prednisone and dexamethasone. Do these sound familiar? In the past, your doctor may have prescribed corticosteroids for you for conditions or illnesses entirely unrelated to cancer, but the dosages were much smaller and the course of treatment much shorter. Some additional chemotherapy drugs that do not fit into any of the listed categories also are available.

Taking heart from new developments

Every day, cancer research moves forward. Here are just a few new developments.

Introducing new drugs

New chemotherapy drugs are being introduced all the time. Of course, all new treatments undergo years of research and testing before the Food and Drug Administration (FDA) releases them for public use. This testing period allows scientists to determine if the drugs work, if they work better than treatments already in use, and if they are safe. Drugs waiting for approval, drugs that are considered experimental, are tested in clinical trials. (For more on clinical trials, see Chapter 6.)

Changing the course of treatment

Other new developments include pairing established drugs with new drugs for a better outcome and administering chemotherapy drugs on a different timetable. Sometimes when the schedule of treatment is altered, the effectiveness of the drug is improved. For that reason, even after chemotherapy drugs are approved by the FDA, the schedule and manner in which the drugs are delivered are explored in clinical trials so the effectiveness of the chemotherapy can be further improved.

Exploring gene therapy

One of the most heartening areas of research is *gene therapy,* which involves introducing genetic material into the body (or directly into the tumor) to fight cancer and improve the performance of the immune system. You remember genes from science class. Our genes, inherited from our parents, make us who we are. A gene, as defined by the National Cancer Institute (NCI), is part of a DNA molecule. We each have between 50,000 and 100,000 genes. Genes carry instructions that allow the cells to produce specific proteins, such as enzymes. During the creation of proteins, cells use another molecule, RNA, to translate the genetic information stored in DNA.

A fact sheet from the NCI explains the following:

> *Only certain genes in a cell are active at any given moment. As cells mature, many genes become permanently inactive. The pattern of active and inactive genes in a cell and the resulting protein composition determine what kind of cell it is and what it can and cannot do. Flaws in genes can result in disease.*

In gene therapy, a carrier known as a *vector* delivers a gene to a cell either in a petri dish in a laboratory or in a person's body. Some of these altered genes are designed to kill cancer cells. Some are designed to enhance the body's receptivity to chemotherapy and radiation. Some are designed to prevent cancer cells from developing new blood vessels. Currently, most vectors are viruses that have been altered to make them safe, though risks still exist. As we write this, gene therapy is available only in clinical trials.

Investigating Different Delivery Systems

Most chemotherapy drugs are delivered directly into a vein, through an intravenous drip. Some are injected into a muscle, under the skin, into spaces around body tissues, or directly into the cancerous masses. Still other chemotherapy drugs come in pill form. Not all chemotherapy drugs are available in all forms of delivery.

Having intravenous chemotherapy

Did you know that some chemotherapy drugs come in big plastic bags? The drugs get out of the bags and into your bloodstream through thin tubes attached to a thin needle that goes into a vein in your body. This delivery system is commonly known as an IV (for *intravenous*) drip. Basically, a chemo nurse or another technician hooks you up, and you sit for a couple of hours or more as the liquid chemotherapy drugs slowly make their way through your body.

Where do you sit? That depends.

Some people are admitted to the hospital for treatment, but most people have chemo at the doctor's office, at an infusion clinic, or in a hospital's out-patient department.

Who decides? Again, that depends. Generally the deciding factors include

- ✔ Your insurance company's rules
- ✔ Your doctor's preference
- ✔ Your preference
- ✔ Your chemotherapy drugs
- ✔ Your general medical condition

For most people, intravenous chemotherapy is a group experience, held in a sun-filled room with large, overstuffed lounge chairs arranged along the wall (see Figure 4-1). Plenty of magazines are on hand, and there may even be a television set with the volume turned to low. Extra chairs are always available for your chemo buddy (see Chapter 8).

One thing you can do for yourself during chemo is drink water. Bring your own bottle, or bring a glass to refill from the office water cooler. Increased intake of water moves the chemotherapy drugs through your system more readily, not to mention all the other benefits of moisturizing from within.

Making new friends at chemo

If you were expecting chemo to be a private, somber experience, well — it ain't necessarily so. Typically, people who already have had a treatment or two greet newcomers and introduce themselves. The next time they see you, they likely will ask how you're doing, and you probably will be moved to ask them the same question. If you're feeling fine, you may strike up a longer conversation. Sometimes, several people share practical tips that make the experience of cancer easier. Other times, they exchange recipes, show off photos of their children, or deliver impromptu book reviews.

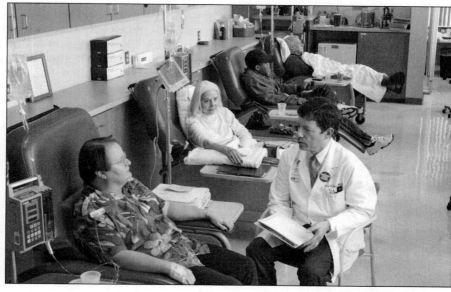

Figure 4-1:
No singers
allowed in
the chemo
lounge, but
chatting and
laughter are
encouraged.

This camaraderie certainly is pleasant, but it also serves to remind you that you're not alone on your journey through cancer.

If you're out of sorts and don't feel like talking the day you come in for chemo, you may choose to just sit quietly with your spouse or friend. Probably, no one will pester you to talk, but if you're feeling pressured to do so and really don't want to, everyone in the room will understand if you simply explain that you want to close your eyes and rest during the treatment. These people all are intimately acquainted with fatigue.

Pass the yams, please

One woman we know was not particularly looking forward to a chemotherapy appointment scheduled the day before Thanksgiving. She knew that her anti-nausea drugs would cause her to feel tired and generally out of sorts for the holiday, which happened to be a favorite of hers. Imagine her surprise when she arrived at the doctor's office and discovered the staff had prepared a complete Thanksgiving dinner for everyone receiving chemotherapy.

This thoughtful — and extremely tasty — gesture changed the entire experience for everyone there.

Considering a catheter

One of the biggest hurdles to a relatively comfortable chemotherapy experience may be the insertion of the IV needle, especially if you're the sort who doesn't have veins that pop up and beg to be stuck. An alternative delivery method is available: a catheter.

A catheter is a thin, flexible tube with one end placed in a large vein inside your body and the other end outside the body (see Figure 4-2). With a catheter, you can receive chemotherapy drugs directly through the tube, and you also can avoid any sticks each time a blood sample is required. Sometimes, the catheter is attached to a small plastic or metal disc placed just under the skin. This disc is called a *port* — simply a recognition that it serves as the entry point for your catheter.

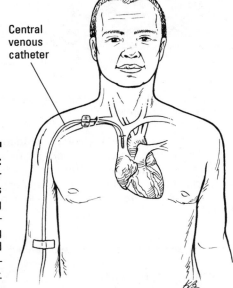

Central venous catheter

Figure 4-2:
A catheter makes taking chemo — and having blood tests — easier.

When you first hear about it, the idea of a catheter may sound intrusive and not particularly pleasant. It may seem like just one more thing that you have to put up with now that you have made room in your life for cancer. If you have this reaction, ask your doctor to show you a catheter so you can see how innocuous it appears. Also, ask if you can meet a person who has a catheter so you can learn more about it from someone with experience. All things considered, a catheter makes chemotherapy easier, and that's good.

If you do choose to have a catheter, a surgeon will put it in place during a short outpatient procedure at a hospital or surgical center. You will be sedated and, therefore, miss the whole thing. The catheter will remain in place until your chemotherapy treatments are over. Then, you will meet the surgeon at the hospital or surgical center again. This time, you likely will be given only local anesthesia — meaning you will be awake — and the catheter will be removed.

If you are the squeamish sort, you may want to close your eyes when the surgeon pulls the catheter from your body. On the other hand, if you watch surgery on television all the time for entertainment, seeing the doctor pull out the tube will be a snap.

After the catheter has been removed, use a small plastic bag filled with frozen peas to help keep down swelling. As a more permanent reminder of the catheter, you will have a 1½-inch scar, but even that will fade with time.

Wearing a pump

Some chemotherapy treatments are delivered by pumps that provide chemo on the go. Generally, a registered nurse who works at your doctor's office or who comes to your home programs the pump so you receive the drugs you need at the prescribed rate. With most pumps, you can have chemo at home, chemo at work, chemo at the ballpark — or wherever you go. When the treatment is finished, a nurse disconnects the pump. Pumps may be used for a few hours daily or for several days in a row — it depends upon the regimen your doctor prescribes for you and your cancer.

Two pump options are available:

- ✔ **Internal:** An internal pump, shaped like a small disk and filled with anticancer drugs, is sometimes used to treat colon cancer that has spread to the liver. First, the pump is inserted under the skin during surgery. A catheter that runs from the pump to the hepatic artery delivers the drugs directly into the liver.

- ✔ **External:** A small, lightweight, battery-powered external pump (see Figure 4-3) is carried in a fanny pack or shoulder pack. The pump is hooked up to an intravenous line so the anticancer drugs may freely flow through the body. Some people wear the pack openly; others wear it underneath their clothing. If you have an external pump, you must protect it from water and avoid bumping it against any hard surfaces.

If the kind of chemotherapy you need is best delivered through a pump, your oncologist or nurse will show you how it works, how to care for it, and what to do if you think the pump isn't working correctly.

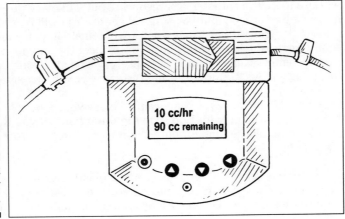

Figure 4-3:
Some external pumps can be carried in a small fanny pack or shoulder pack.

10 cc/hr
90 cc remaining

Taking chemotherapy by mouth

Some chemotherapy drugs are available as pills or capsules, or in liquid form. Researchers know that many people find the idea of taking chemotherapy by mouth very appealing, and new drugs are under development all the time.

The issue of compliance comes into play with this type of delivery system. Doctors consider people *compliant* if they do what they are told, but (of course) not everyone does everything that the doctor says to do. Even people with every intention of exhibiting compliance may forget to take a chemotherapy pill, which could affect the results of the treatment, either in the short-term or the long-term.

Talk to your doctor about whether your chemotherapy drugs can be taken by mouth.

Looking at lesser-known forms of chemotherapy

Some lesser-known forms of chemotherapy also are available. Your doctor will let you know if your particular situation would be best served by one of these options:

✔ **Injection chemotherapy:** A few chemotherapy drugs are administered by injection into a muscle, under the skin, or directly into a cancerous area of the skin.

✔ **Intrathecal chemotherapy:** Sometimes used for cancer in the central nervous system, intrathecal chemotherapy is delivered into the spinal fluid through a needle placed in the spinal column.

✔ **Intraperitoneal chemotherapy:** With this method, anticancer drugs are delivered through a catheter into the abdomen.

✔ **Topical chemotherapy:** Some chemotherapy drugs are available in creams or lotions that are applied directly to the skin.

Evaluating Your Oncologist's Recommendation

After your diagnosis has been made and your test results are available, your oncologist likely will recommend that you proceed with chemotherapy — as long as she truly believes that it will help you. Before you begin chemotherapy, you'll receive a treatment plan, your optimum drug dosage will be determined, and you may want to get a second opinion.

Setting up a treatment plan

Your oncologist will present you with a treatment plan that she believes is best for you. That plan likely will include the following elements:

✔ Information about the prognosis for your kind and stage of cancer

✔ A recommendation for a specific combination of chemotherapy drugs

✔ A method of delivery for those drugs and a location for treatments

✔ A schedule for the frequency and length of treatment

✔ Recommendations for scans or other tests to determine the effect of treatments as they progress

✔ Information on drugs or treatments to help your body better withstand chemotherapy

✔ Information on clinical trials that you may want to consider joining

The plan will be based on several factors, including

✔ The kind of cancer you have

✔ The stage and grade of your cancer

> ✔ Your age
>
> ✔ Your overall health
>
> ✔ Your personal circumstances, such as how far you live from a treatment center, your ability to travel, the availability of help at home, the demands of your job, and your family responsibilities

The treatment plan your doctor designs for you also will be based on the experiences of others who have had the same kind of cancer, the results of recent research, and the availability of a clinical trial that your doctor thinks is promising for you. (For more on clinical trials, see Chapter 6.) That said, your doctor will take your individual circumstances into account, and the plan will be tailor-made for you.

Determining the dose

Your treatment plan is based in part on the stage of your cancer (see Chapter 3). After the stage has been determined, a nationally accepted set of standards for treatment is followed. (The standards and the doses of the drugs are determined in clinical trials.)

Maybe you think you would prefer larger doses of the drugs so you could get treatment over with sooner. That's not a good idea. Even though large doses of the drugs can kill more cancer cells than small doses, large doses of these powerful drugs also can produce more debilitating side effects (see Chapters 10 and 11).

Faith in the process

Baseball player Eric Davis was diagnosed with colon cancer in May of 1997. He had surgery in June, and the doctor removed a tumor the size of an orange. In his autobiography, *Born to Play* (Penguin), Davis writes about not wanting to go to chemotherapy. He tells about his doubts that the chemo was working.

A young girl, who also was going through chemotherapy, asked Davis why he thought the anticancer drugs weren't working. Touched by the girl's question, Davis changed his thinking. He decided to believe that the chemotherapy was working, and he finished all 46 treatments.

Today, when people tell Davis that he was courageous for undergoing the treatment, he replies, "I didn't do anything that any other self-respecting human being wouldn't do — and that was fight for life." He always adds, "I couldn't have done it alone."

What did he learn from cancer? "Well," says Davis, "I never put off anything until tomorrow."

Most doctors recommend a maximum dose that is considered safe, and then they work to offset the more serious aspects of the side effects. Also, the doses for some drugs are adjusted based on your height, weight, and/or age. Of course, the most important determinant of the dose of chemotherapy that you receive is your tolerance to the dose that your doctor prescribes.

What matters most, of course, to all parties concerned, is that the chemotherapy works and that you survive your treatment with few (ideally, no) long-term negative effects.

Getting a second opinion

If you seek a second opinion, you present two trained professionals with all the facts about your situation, from the diagnosis to the recommended treatment plan, and compare what they say. The doctors may agree, which should boost your confidence about the plan. The doctors may not agree, in which case you need to understand exactly what the points of disagreement are in order to make the best decision.

Whether you get a second opinion may be up to you, or it may be a decision that your insurance company makes for you. Some insurance companies require a second opinion. Even those that don't require it may pay for a visit with another physician if you choose to get another opinion. Before you seek a second opinion, check with your insurance company. (But then you probably already knew that.)

If you are unsure where to go for a second opinion, consider these options:

- Ask your doctor to recommend another oncologist.
- Call another doctor on your insurance plan.
- Call a nearby hospital or medical school.
- Check with the Cancer Information Service (800-422-6237), a service of the National Cancer Institute.
- Ask a friend or co-worker who has been treated for cancer.

Sometimes, in the course of seeking a second opinion, you may meet a doctor who, for any number of reasons, appeals to you more than the oncologist you originally had chosen. If that happens and you are confused whether to switch doctors, remember to think of yourself as a consumer of healthcare. You have the right to spend your money with a doctor who makes you feel confident and comfortable, so if you want to make a change, do so.

Searching for Dr. Right

You can't overestimate the importance of having a good oncologist on your side. But *good* doesn't just mean educated, informed, and able to identify your best treatment options. A good oncologist — one with or without a charismatic bedside manner — sees you as an individual and encourages you to take an active role in your treatment and recovery.

So how do you know when you've found the right doctor?

✔ You know you have a good doctor when that doctor recommends that you buy a small notebook and write down your questions between visits so everything that concerns you can be addressed.

✔ You know you have a good doctor when that doctor encourages you to call the office any time things are not going the way you think they should.

✔ You know you have a good doctor when that doctor provides information on clinical trials in which you can participate to help yourself, as well as others who may have the same kind of cancer.

✔ And you know you have a good doctor when that doctor recommends that you get a second opinion on your diagnosis and your treatment plan before proceeding.

Changing doctors is a business decision, not a personal one, even if your reasons for wanting to change strike you as personal.

When you have returned to your original oncologist or made the decision to switch, you can start attending to the details of your treatment.

Making the Best Choice for You

In some instances, your treatment plan may include specific choices. For instance, there may be two types of treatment that work especially well for the kind of cancer that you have. One anticancer drug may be administered over a shorter period of time and cause more troubling side effects than the second option, which may require a longer treatment period. Your doctor should present all the pros and cons and give you a few days to make the decision.

If you are comfortable deciding after you have read all the material you have been given and had all your questions answered, so be it. If you don't want the responsibility of deciding, you can always ask the doctor which treatment he would choose for a family member. That sounds like a trick question, but it isn't, so ask away.

Asking the right questions

At this point, you will have lots of questions. One particularly difficult question is whether you choose to proceed with chemotherapy at all. For most people, the answer to that question is a no-brainer. No one wants to have chemotherapy, of course, but people who hope that it will kill their cancer choose it. For others, the answer may be influenced by religious or philosophical beliefs, and they may choose not to move forward. That decision creates a difficult situation for the doctor, who is left holding a discarded solution to a very serious problem.

If you do decide to proceed with chemotherapy, some of your questions at this point will be specific and have to do with the near future. Some of the questions will be more general and deal with the months, even years, to come. Your doctor should be able to answer some of the specific questions, but only time will answer some of the others.

For instance, you may want to know right now whether chemotherapy will make you ill and, if so, how ill, and what can be done if that happens. The doctor likely will be able to answer only the last part of that question. We've said it before and will say it again: Going through cancer treatments is different for everyone. Not only that, but the second round of chemotherapy may affect you differently than the first and third. No one can predict exactly what will happen.

Still, you can ask — and ask often — what may happen and what you can expect as you go through chemotherapy. And at every step along the way, you can ask why you are experiencing certain side effects and what to do about them. (For specific information on side effects from chemotherapy, see Chapters 10 and 11.)

You can ask about any weekly or monthly tumor board meetings or "cancer conferences" held at the medical center that your medical team plans to have about your treatment. You can ask about your team's continuing education programs and what efforts will be made to keep you up-to-date on current research. Frankly, you can ask whatever comes to mind.

Getting the right answers

Be relentless in your questioning of your doctor or nurse, and be comfortable with that role. Some patients consider asking questions to be a challenge to the doctor's authority, but asking questions about your healthcare actually allows you to be an active part of your survival team. (For more on putting together a survival team, see Part V of this book.)

When you make decisions with your doctor about your treatment, you feel more involved in the process. That involvement provides you with an element of control in a period of your life when you probably feel very much out of control. Cancer comes unbidden, and it changes everything. You can't control that, but you can feel that you have some say about your treatment and your quality of life during treatment.

Moving forward with confidence

From the moment that you learn of your diagnosis to the moment that you sit in the oncologist's office and devise a treatment plan, only a short period of time passes. In a matter of days, you're thrown into a new culture and taught a new language, and your head is spinning, your mind in a whirl. Yet, you know that every decision you make likely will affect the rest of your life.

As you get ready to implement your treatment plan, you may be inclined to panic, but we strongly recommend against it.

This is a good time to remind yourself that you have learned what you need to know for now, if not more, and that you have consulted with people who know more about this new culture and this new language than you. Together, you have made a plan based on the facts available, and you are aware that it can be altered to serve you better as you go along. The real beauty of the plan is that it is in place. Questions have been asked, questions have been answered, and now you have a place to begin.

At some point (the sooner the better), you will be ready to take the next step. That step begins with a deep breath and builds to the place where you achieve a sense of calm, a mood of quiet confidence.

How is that possible? Remind yourself that you have made the best choices possible based on the best knowledge available at this time. Remind yourself that you have a plan and that you'll continue to learn more with each day that passes.

You can use this sense of calm, this confidence, to help quiet your fears and prepare you for the future.

One thing is for certain. You are not alone on your journey through cancer.

Chapter 5

Defining Radiation: A Burning Issue

*R*adiation therapy is a *local,* or site-specific, treatment for cancer. Radiation may shrink or eradicate tumors, and it kills cancer cells that may linger after a tumor has been removed surgically.

The idea of radiation may seem otherworldly, like something that would be available in the future in a galaxy far, far away. Actually, radiation has been used to treat cancer and other diseases for more than 100 years. Three discoveries, all of which occurred in the years just preceding 1900, led to radiation therapy: x-rays, radioactivity, and radium. In the early years of the 20th century, surgeons typically administered a single massive blast of radiation to a patient's body. Sometimes, miraculously, that worked — but often these earliest treatments were not successful.

That was then. This is now. Sophisticated machines deliver carefully calibrated doses of external beam radiation to a precise site anywhere in the body. Another form of radiation therapy, called *brachytherapy,* uses radioactive wires, seeds, or rods that are placed in the body close to the site of the tumor or directly into it. Today, between 50 and 60 percent of all cancer patients undergo some form of radiation therapy. Science, as they say, marches on.

Let's have a hand for Madame Curie

We can thank Marie and Pierre Curie for helping develop what we now know as radiation therapy and for founding the Radium Institute (now the Curie Institute) in Paris. Marie actually coined the word *radioactivity* in 1898. Though she worked at a time when women's contributions in science often were unrecognized, Curie was the first woman to receive the Nobel Prize, which she won twice, in 1903 and 1911.

Most of us learned in school to call this distinguished scientist "Madame Curie," but few people recall that she was born Marya Sklodowska in Poland. In France, her adopted country, Curie was lauded as a national hero for fearlessly driving an x-ray truck right to the front lines during World War I. Curie died at 66 of a rare leukemia, which probably can be traced to her work. Legend has it that radioactive dust was found years later on her personal cookbooks.

That dust also was found on her scientific papers and personal journals, but after those materials were treated and declared safe, author Barbara Goldsmith was among the first to peruse them. The result was her highly acclaimed book, issued in 2004, titled *Obsessive Genius: The Inner World of Marie Curie* (W.W. Norton & Co.).

The job of radiation therapy is to cure or control cancer, a disease that kills 1,500 Americans every day, according to the National Cancer Institute. One big reason more people *don't* die of cancer is the effectiveness of radiation treatments. The idea of radiation therapy can be scary, but the reality is that this time-tested form of treatment is powerful and offers hope to people with cancer.

In this chapter, we introduce you to different forms of radiation therapy, describe the team of specialists who will provide the therapy, and offer guidelines on working with your doctor throughout therapy.

Understanding Radiation Therapy

Radiation therapy takes place at a hospital on an outpatient basis under the direction of a radiation oncologist and a radiation oncology team. (Chapter 12 describes the experience of undergoing radiation therapy.) Radiation therapy does produce side effects at the site under treatment, which we discuss in detail in Chapter 13, but many people undergoing radiation therapy have little difficulty maintaining their regular daily schedules.

That's not always the case for people who undergo radiation therapy and chemotherapy at the same time. Sometimes, both therapies are indicated simultaneously because of the likelihood of a better outcome.

Figure 5-1 shows what a CT image of cancer looks like before and after radiation therapy.

Figure 5-1:
These CT
images
show a
patient
before (left)
and after
(right)
radiation
therapy.

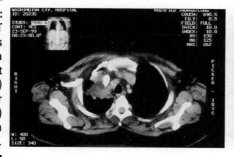 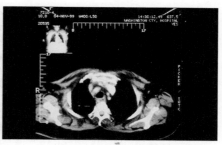

Source: Missouri Baptist Medical Center

There are two main types of radiation therapy: External beam radiation, also known as *teletherapy,* and internal radiation therapy, or *brachytherapy.* Which type is most appropriate for you? That depends on these factors:

✔ The kind of cancer you have

✔ The stage or grade of your tumor

✔ Whether your doctor has recommended surgery in conjunction with other treatments

Sometimes, both kinds of radiation treatments are used together to treat cancer — external beam radiation to destroy cancerous cells in the area surrounding the tumor, and internal radiation therapy to deliver a higher dose of radiation at the exact site of the tumor.

Of the two, external beam radiation — used to treat cancers of the head and neck area, breast, lung, colon, and prostate — is the more common, so we'll start there.

Defining external radiation therapy

In Chapter 2, we mention that cancer routinely is portrayed as an enemy — rightly so, because it can kill you — and most of the language used to describe how cancer treatments work is harsh and makes use of military imagery. Following our military metaphor, external beam radiation therapy mounts the assault five days a week, usually for six or seven weeks — a timeline designed to keep the enemy on the run. (See Chapter 12 for information on setting up your treatment schedule.) Like chemotherapy, this type of radiation therapy is a cumulative process, with every treatment building on the last one.

Going through external beam radiation therapy is a lot like getting a routine x-ray: You feel nothing, and you see nothing. You do, however, hear something — the buzzing and clicking of the machine that delivers the radiation to the cancer site.

Most often, the machine used during external radiation therapy is a linear accelerator (*LINAC* for short). A time-tested machine that is updated as improvements are developed, the *LINAC* can deliver beams of both low- and high-energy photons and electrons. Other machines used in external beam radiation therapy include orthovoltage x-ray machines and cobalt-60 machines, which deliver low-energy beams.

Several different types of external beam radiation are available, which we explain in the following sections. Keep in mind that the necessary equipment is not always available in smaller hospitals. To get the treatment you need, you may have to travel to a medical center that has the up-to-date, high-tech equipment required.

Photon/electron radiation therapy

The most common form of radiation therapy in use is high-energy photon (x-ray) beam radiation, which is used to destroy or shrink tumors and to destroy any cancer cells in an area where a tumor has been removed. Most cancers are treated with high-energy photon radiation. Low-energy radiation is used to treat surface tumors.

Electrons are charged particles used to treat more superficial tumor sites, such as lymph nodes in the neck; to boost treatment of a breast cancer site; or to treat skin cancers. Electron beams have different energies and must be carefully chosen for the appropriate depth of the cancer being treated.

Often, patients are treated with a combination of photons (x-rays) and electrons (accelerated charged particles).

Three-dimensional conformal radiation therapy (3D-CRT)

This treatment sounds like a cousin of one of the *Star Wars* androids, doesn't it? It isn't. Three-dimensional conformal radiation therapy calls on computers and computer-assisted tomography scans (also know as CT or CAT scans), along with magnetic resonance imaging scans (MR or MRI scans), to create a three-dimensional representation of a tumor and the surrounding organs. Tools called *multileaf collimators,* or *blocks,* match the radiation beams to the size and shape of the tumor. This allows for less radiation exposure to nearby normal tissue.

Intensity modulated radiation therapy (IMRT)

This type of radiation therapy is a form of 3D-CRT that breaks the radiation beam into many small "beamlets," with individually adjusted levels of intensity. Sometimes, IMRT can be used to deliver a higher dose of radiation directly to the tumor while limiting radiation received by normal tissues. This currently is the most precise, cutting-edge form of external radiation, and it requires meticulous planning and quality assurance on the part of the radiation oncologist, physicist, dosimetrist, and radiation therapists.

Proton beam radiation therapy

Proton beam therapy uses protons (charged particles), rather than x-rays, to treat cancer. Proton therapy provides a sharper beam, which may be useful in treating lesions close to the spinal cord, for example. However, there's a price to pay for that precision: potentially intensified side effects. This therapy is very costly, and few proton beam therapy machines are available in the United States.

Neutron beam radiation therapy

Some tumors that are *radio-resistant,* or difficult to kill with conventional radiation therapy, can be treated with neutron beam therapy. This type of therapy occasionally is used to treat some inoperable tumors, though most often such tumors are treated with radiation therapy using photon (x-ray) and electron radiation therapy.

Stereotactic radiation therapy

In stereotactic radiation therapy, high doses of radiation are focused on a small area, no larger than 2 to 3 centimeters. Also, many beams of high-dose radiation converge on the tumor from different directions. This therapy is often used to treat small tumors in the head, brain, lungs, and other sites.

Defining internal radiation therapy

Internal radiation therapy, or *brachytherapy,* is an inside job, so to speak. In this method of therapy, radioactive material in small sealed containers is implanted near or at the tumor site. The radioactive material, known as *isotopes,* comes in wires, ribbons, capsules (called *seeds;* see Figure 5-2), or rods.

Brachytherapy is used to treat a number of different cancers, including cancers of the

- Anus
- Bladder

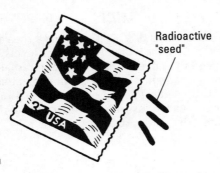

Radioactive "seed"

Figure 5-2:
Radioactive seeds used in brachytherapy are quite small.

- Brain
- Breast
- Cervix
- Esophagus
- Eye
- Head and neck
- Lung
- Prostate
- Rectum
- Skin
- Uterus
- Vagina

With some types of brachytherapy, some isotopes remain in the body long after the radiation has been expended and the sources are no longer radioactive. Other isotopes, placed inside the body only temporarily, are removed after the tumor has received the prescribed dose of radiation. It all depends on the specific type of brachytherapy you receive. We describe the common types in the following sections.

Interstitial brachytherapy

This type of therapy involves implanting radioactive seeds, rods, or wires in the area of a tumor or a cancerous prostate. These isotopes, or radioactive sources, may be inserted and removed on the same day and then reinserted within 36 to 48 hours. Sometimes, they stay in the body permanently. Common sites treated with interstitial brachytherapy include head and neck, skin, breast, prostate, soft tissues, and pelvis.

Partial breast irradiation

A form of brachytherapy known as *partial breast irradiation* offers promise for the future, though the treatment is not considered standard care at this time. Partial breast irradiation requires only one week of radiation for women who have undergone a lumpectomy for breast cancer, compared to the standard six or seven weeks of external beam radiation. At this point, some studies five years after treatment have produced what doctors call "acceptable results." More studies are underway.

To track the effect of interstitial brachytherapy on a man treated for prostate cancer, see Figure 5-3. The chart measures prostate specific antigen (PSA) levels before and after radiation therapy. Once used primarily to determine whether cancer treatments were working, the PSA test — a blood test — now also is used to screen for and diagnose prostate cancer.

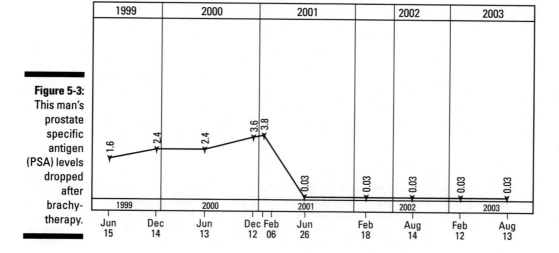

Figure 5-3: This man's prostate specific antigen (PSA) levels dropped after brachytherapy.

Intracavitary brachytherapy

This type of therapy is used to irradiate the walls of a cavity in the body or nearby tissue. The isotopes are put in place with an applicator. After the tumor has received the prescribed dose of radiation, the applicator is removed. This therapy typically is used to treat gynecological cancers, as well as cancers of the esophagus and lungs.

Systemic radiation therapy

Some radioactive isotopes can be swallowed, given intravenously, or administered by injection to deliver *systemic treatment* — treatment that spreads throughout the body via the bloodstream. For instance, some patients with some types of thyroid cancer may be asked to swallow radioactive iodine capsules. Also, patients with metastatic cancer to the bone may be treated with intravenous liquid radioisotopes such as Strontium-89 or Samarium-153 deposited in the affected bone cells.

Intraoperative radiation therapy

Sometimes, a radiation oncologist delivers radiation therapy during surgery. This type of therapy is used when a tumor is dangerously close to healthy organs. The surgeon moves the healthy organs aside so that the tumor can receive radiation therapy.

Radioimmunotherapy

In Chapter 2, we explain that the body is capable of making antibodies in response to the presence of *antigens,* which are shreds of viruses and other foreign substances that invade the body. Here, the focus is tumor antigens.

Some types of antibodies can be manufactured in a laboratory and then attached to radioactive isotopes to combat the tumor antigens. The antibodies are injected into the body, where they circulate in the bloodstream, hunting for cancer cells. The radiation in the antibodies destroys the invading cells. This therapy — known in the media as *liquid radiation* — is used to treat patients with certain types of lymphomas that test positive for tumor antigens. Other tumor sites eventually may be treated with radioimmunotherapy as further studies uncover other tumor antigens to be targeted.

Investigational radiation therapies

Several additional types of experimental radiation therapy are available in just a few medical centers, where the treatments are under study to determine how they can best help people with cancer. Studies currently in progress include evaluations of the combination of different chemotherapy drugs concurrently and/or sequentially with radiation therapy for lung, pancreas, stomach, brain, breast, and other cancers. Another focus of radiation research includes different regimens of radiation therapy delivered in a shorter period (higher daily dose) versus a more protracted course (lower daily dose).

Several studies are looking at the molecular/cellular level to increase the attack on the tumor and lessen treatment side effects in head and neck, lung, and gastrointestinal malignancies. Also, several studies are adding chemotherapy to radiation, looking for higher cure rates but also evaluating the side effects of combined modality. Expect to hear more about these therapies in the years to come.

Exploring ways to improve radiation therapy treatments

Additional treatment options, some of them experimental, are sometimes made available to people undergoing radiation therapy. Here are brief descriptions of two drugs used as "helpers," most often in external beam radiation therapy:

- *Radiosensitizers* are drugs designed to make tumors more sensitive to radiation, which, in turn, may help radiation do a better job at destroying tumors.

- *Radioprotectors* are drugs that researchers hope will do a better job of protecting normal tissues near an area undergoing radiation therapy.

Evaluating Your Radiation Oncologist's Recommendation

At this point, you may be suffering from information overload and wondering whether you need to know all this.

Not really.

Technically, all you need to know is what form of radiation therapy your doctor recommends and why. Some people don't want even that much information, but others want to do independent research in order to learn as much as they can about cancer and cancer treatments. You know which kind of person you are, and you will act accordingly. Your doctor will make a recommendation for treatment after your diagnosis has been determined and all your test results are available.

Setting up a treatment plan

Your treatment plan will be based on several factors, including

- The kind of cancer you have
- The stage and grade of your cancer

- ✔ Your age
- ✔ Your overall health
- ✔ Your personal circumstances, such as how far you live from a treatment center, your ability to travel, the availability of help at home, the demands of your job, and your family responsibilities

The treatment plan your doctor designs for you also will be based on the experiences of others who have had the same kind of cancer, the results of recent research, and the availability of a clinical trial that your doctor thinks is promising for you. (For more on clinical trials, see Chapter 6.) That said, your doctor will take your individual circumstances into account, and the plan will be tailor-made for you.

Throughout your treatment, your doctor will monitor and evaluate your body's response to radiation therapy. If you do well with radiation therapy, your treatments will take place according to schedule, following logically from the first to the last. However, if radiation therapy is particularly tough for you, your doctor may spread out the treatments or perhaps halt therapy altogether.

Only time will tell.

Determining the dose

Before your treatments begin, your radiation oncologist and a team of specialists will determine the right dose of radiation for you — a dose that will deliver the maximum amount required to damage and kill cancer cells while minimally affecting healthy cells. If you have had surgery and your tumor has been removed, the dose of radiation therapy will be calibrated to treat a specific area where the tumor once was. If the tumor has not been removed, the following factors will help determine what dose is right for you:

- ✔ The type of tumor
- ✔ The size of the tumor
- ✔ The grade and stage of the tumor
- ✔ The proximity of the tumor to healthy tissue

Of course, what matters most to all parties concerned is that the radiation therapy works and that you survive your treatment with few (ideally, no) long-term negative effects.

Meeting the team

When it comes to radiation therapy, there are a lot of concerned parties. The number of people on your team is actually quite impressive! We've already said that a radiation oncologist will direct your treatment. Throughout, he will maintain contact with your medical oncologist.

Radiation oncologists have extensive training in the safe use of radiation. The American Board of Radiology certifies those doctors who pass a special examination in this field. You want to ask if your doctor is board-certified.

Here are some of the other specialists who will work with you:

- **Medical radiation physicists:** These trained specialists work with your radiation oncologist during the planning and delivery of your treatment. They make certain that your treatment is tailored precisely for you. They also develop and direct quality-control programs for equipment and procedures, and they regularly perform safety tests on the equipment.

- **Dosimetrists:** These trained technicians work with your radiation oncologist and the medical physicists to calculate the dose required to treat you.

- **Radiation therapists:** These board-certified trained technicians work with your radiation oncologist to administer your treatment. They keep daily records and also routinely check the equipment to make sure it is working correctly.

- **Radiation oncology nurses:** These specially trained registered nurses help care for you and your family during consultation, while you receive treatment, and throughout your follow-up care. Radiation oncology nurses are always available to talk with you about side effects, help you manage those side effects, and answer any questions about your treatment.

Getting a second opinion

In Chapter 4, we explain why you may want to seek a second opinion regarding a chemotherapy treatment plan. The same advice applies if you're facing radiation therapy. Take a good look at that information, and consider whether your comfort level will increase if you get feedback from another doctor about what's best for you.

Making the Best Choice for You

After you've settled on a radiation oncologist, you can turn your attention to your treatment plan. At the end of Chapter 4, where we discuss chemotherapy, we explain the importance of asking the right questions of your doctor and being relentless in your pursuit of answers. The same advice applies if you're facing radiation therapy, so we recommend taking a good look at those suggestions.

One of your questions likely will be whether radiation therapy will cause debilitating side effects, and if so, what can be done. The radiation oncologist likely will be able to answer only the last part of that question. Most side effects from radiation therapy — which we discuss in Chapter 13 — occur at the site of the therapy, usually about halfway through treatment. Many of the side effects can be treated effectively. We've said it before and we'll say it again: Going through cancer treatments is different for everyone. No one can predict exactly what will happen.

Chapter 6

Setting New Standards: The Role of Clinical Trials

. . . .

In This Chapter

▶ Exploring the purpose of clinical trials

▶ Understanding the three phases of clinical trials

▶ Pondering the benefits and risks

▶ Knowing what questions to ask

▶ Taking part in a clinical trial

. . . .

*E*very day, in many parts of the world, researchers are working to find better treatments for cancer. Some of these efforts take place in laboratories. Some experimental treatments are being tested on a small number of people who have not had success with standard treatments. Some experimental treatments that have proven to be effective on a small number of people now are being tested on larger numbers of people.

These tests, called *clinical trials,* represent the future of cancer treatment. Every standard treatment in use today originally was tested in clinical trials.

Clinical trials are not for everyone. For that matter, clinical trials are not available to everyone. In this chapter, we discuss the nature of clinical trials and offer some guidance to help you decide if you would like to take part.

Grasping the Importance of Clinical Trials

Research studies in all fields of medicine are known as clinical trials. These studies are conducted with an eye to the future, in hopes of finding safer or more effective methods to screen for, prevent, diagnose, or treat a variety of diseases.

Realizing the scope of cancer trials

Just how many clinical trials on cancer are there? Here's some perspective: In June 2004, more than 25,000 cancer specialists attended the conference for the American Society of Clinical Oncologists. At that conference, participants could learn about the results of 3,700 different cancer research studies.

These studies — and others in related fields — are conducted on many fronts. For example, many cancer research studies address the following areas:

- New techniques for screening for, diagnosing, or staging cancer
- New anticancer drugs
- New methods of surgery
- New approaches to radiation therapy
- New combinations of standard treatments
- New technologies, such as gene therapy

Tests are carried out according to standard procedures used to evaluate new drugs and methods of treatment. (Read more about these procedures in the next section.) Powerful treatments in use today for breast cancer, colon cancer, rectal cancer, and childhood cancers all began in clinical trials. The results of clinical trials have allowed many people with cancer to live longer, and these scientific tests also have pointed the way to future research.

Understanding the development of clinical trials

A clinical trial is not the first step in the development of a new drug or treatment. In fact, it is one of the last. Research and development generally begins in a scientific laboratory. After extensive testing, scientists may test a promising drug or technique on animals. Later, a small number of volunteers willing to undergo experimental treatments takes part in studies. Based on the results of these studies, drugs and treatments that have been shown to be effective are made available for larger clinical trials.

According to the National Cancer Institute, which is part of the National Institutes of Health, cancer clinical trials include research at three different phases, each designed to answer different questions about the new treatment or technique.

The first two phases generally are made available only to a limited number of patients who are not benefiting from standard treatment.

Here are the three phases of research:

- **Phase I:** This is the first step in testing a new treatment on humans. Researchers may study whether the best way to give a new treatment is by mouth, IV drip, or injection. They may try to determine the best dose and how many times a drug or treatment should be given each day. They also watch for harmful side effects.

- **Phase II:** Trials conducted in Phase II determine whether the new treatment has an anticancer effect. For instance, does the treatment shrink tumors? What types of tumors does it shrink? Does it improve the results of blood tests for some cancers but not others?

- **Phase III:** After a treatment has demonstrated promising results in Phases I and II, Phase III studies compare the results of people taking standard treatments for specific cancers in specific stages with people taking the new treatment. Researchers all over the country conduct Phase III clinical trials, and thousands of people take part.

In Phase III clinical trials, participants are assigned at random to receive either the new treatment or a standard cancer treatment. Participants in clinical trials are divided into the two groups to help avoid bias. In this instance, *bias* is defined as an effect on the results of the study due to personal choices. In most cases, the *treatment group* receives the drug or method being tested, and the *control group* receives a time-tested standard treatment for cancer. All patients, of course, are carefully monitored.

In *single blind* studies, participants are unaware of which group they are in. In *double blind* studies — which are not done in the majority of cases — neither the participant nor the doctor knows whether the participant is in the experimental group or the control group (the group receiving standard treatment). These studies are designed to protect against bias, because participants (and their doctors) may act differently if they know whether they are taking the experimental drug or receiving standard treatment.

Ahoy there, limey!

Though the purpose of clinical trials is to find something new, something better, the use of clinical trials is far from new. One of the first medical research studies on record took place at sea in May of 1747. Aboard a British naval ship called the *Salisbury*, one Dr. James Lind had available to him 12 seamen with scurvy, which we now know is a deficiency of vitamin C. Lind fed them all the same three meals each day but devised six different treatments for the men, whom he divided into pairs. Not surprisingly, the two men who ate oranges and lemons for six days fared the best. In 1754, Lind wrote of his experiment in "A Treatise on Scurvy."

Though Dr. James Lind's experiment on board the H.M.S. *Salisbury* proved that eating oranges and lemons could stave off scurvy, the British Navy dallied for a full 40 years before issuing an order requiring that lemon juice be a standard supply on ships. Once they did that, scurvy was no longer a problem aboard ship, and the number of sick sailors was cut in half.

Because lemons were expensive, over time the Navy switched to limes. And that, dear reader, is the reason that British sailors for so long were referred to as *limeys*.

Comparing the results of two different treatments for the same type of cancer allows researchers to document the study results and show which treatment is more effective and has fewer side effects.

A small number of clinical trials involve the use of placebos for participants in the control group. *Placebos* are pills or injections that look like the drug or substance being tested but contain no drug. Everyone participating is informed if placebos are in use. Again, most clinical trials do not use placebos, and only if a patient agrees to participate in a placebo-controlled clinical trial can she receive a placebo.

Deciding Whether to Participate

The process of deciding whether to take part in a clinical trial may not be a simple one. There are benefits and drawbacks. Asking "What's in it for me?" is entirely legitimate, as your health — maybe your life — is at stake. In other words, if ever a decision called for careful consideration, this is it. Before you decide, take time to consider the benefits and the risks.

Considering the benefits

Here are some of the benefits of clinical trials you should be aware of:

- **Receiving high-quality care:** Everyone participating in a clinical trial receives high-quality cancer care. Some participants receive the new drug or treatment, and others receive the best standard treatment available. The standard treatment may be as good as — or even better than — the new treatment.

- **Benefiting first:** If you are part of the treatment group and the new treatment is found to be successful, you will be among the first to benefit. You also will be informed promptly of any information that comes from the trial that is important to your care.

- **Getting extra attention:** When you participate in a clinical trial, additional people — some of them monitoring the results of the trial on a national basis — look through your records, watching for details that may be important to your care. This administrative oversight may lead to suggestions or even directives to your doctor that may improve the outcome of your treatment.

- **Taking an active role:** The act of investigating what clinical trials are available indicates that you are taking an active role in choosing the best care as you are treated for cancer.

- **Helping others:** Participation in clinical trials improves cancer treatments, offering new hope to future patients — including (potentially) your family members or friends who may develop cancer in the future.

Considering the risks

There are some risks associated with participating in a clinical trial, including the following:

- **Experiencing unexpected side effects:** New treatments may cause unexpected side effects or side effects that are worse than those from standard treatment.

- **Failing to benefit from a new treatment:** Not every participant in a treatment group benefits. Of course, this is also true for some participants in the control group, who may not benefit from standard treatments.

- **Being part of the control group:** The new drug or technique being tested may be more effective than standard treatment, but participants in the control group will not see those benefits.

> ✔ **Taking a financial risk:** Health insurance coverage of clinical trials varies according to the health plan and the study. You should definitely ask at the research office about necessary coverage before calling your insurance company.

Asking questions

Before deciding to take part in a clinical trial, you will have an opportunity to speak with your doctor and the staff conducting the study. This is an opportunity to ask any questions you may have.

This is no time to keep quiet because you think a question may sound silly or make you look foolish. Ask every question on your mind, and if you don't understand a particular answer, ask for clarification. Consider jotting your questions in a notebook and making notes on the answers you receive so you can refer to your written records later.

The National Cancer Institute, a program of the federal government, has outlined suggestions for the types of questions you should ask before deciding to participate in a clinical trial. These questions fall into five categories:

> ✔ Questions about the study:
>
> > • What is the purpose of the study? In what phase is the study?
> >
> > • Why do researchers believe the new treatment being tested may be effective? Has it been tested before?
> >
> > • Who sponsors the study? Who has reviewed it? Who has approved it?
> >
> > • How are the study data and patient safety being checked?
> >
> > • When and where will study results and information go?
>
> ✔ Questions about possible risks and benefits:
>
> > • What are the possible short- and long-term risks, side effects, and benefits to me?
> >
> > • Are there standard treatments for my type of cancer?
> >
> > • How do the possible risks, side effects, and benefits in this study compare with standard treatment?
>
> ✔ Questions about your care:
>
> > • What kind of treatments, medical tests, or procedures will I have during the study? Will they be painful? How do they compare with what I would receive outside the study?

- How often and for how long will I receive the treatment, and how long will I need to remain in the study? Will there be a follow-up after the study?

- Where will my treatment take place? Will I have to be in the hospital at any time? If so, how often and for how long?

- How will I know if the treatment is working?

- Will I be able to see my own doctor? Who will be in charge of my care?

✔ Questions about personal issues:

- How could this study affect my daily life?

- Can you put me in touch with other people who are in the study?

- What support is available for me and my family in the community?

✔ Questions about costs:

- Will I have to pay for any treatment or tests? Will there be other charges?

- What is my health insurance likely to cover?

- Who can help answer any questions for my insurance company or managed-care plan?

Seeking more information

For more information on clinical trials, you may want to ask your doctor for a copy of the National Cancer Institute's booklet called "Taking Part in Clinical Trials: What Cancer Patients Need to Know."

If you want to contact the National Cancer Institute (NCI) directly, you can call 1-800-4-CANCER (1-800-422-6237) or go to the Web sites at http://cancertrials.nci.nih.gov or http://cancernet.nci.nih.gov. In addition to the booklet on clinical trials, the NCI also has videos and CD-ROMs available, some in both English and Spanish.

Other resources for information on clinical trials include the following:

✔ **The Coalition of National Cancer Cooperative Groups:** 877-520-4457 or www.cancertrialshelp.org

✔ **The National Surgical Adjuvant Bowel and Breast Project:** 412-330-4600 or www.nsabp.pitt.edu

✔ **The Radiation Therapy Oncology Group:** 800-227-5463 ext. 4189 or www.rtog.org

Taking Part in a Clinical Trial

Clinical trials take place in cancer centers, hospitals, clinics, and doctors' offices. Taking part may require more tests and visits to the doctor than are required for other patients. As part of the trial, you may be asked to meet with nurses, social workers, and other health professionals in addition to the doctor. You also may be asked to keep a journal or fill out forms tracking your progress.

In any case, you will be told exactly what is expected of you. Every clinical trial has a protocol, or action plan, prepared by the study's investigator, who usually is a doctor. The protocol defines the purpose of the study and why it is being done. The protocol also explains how many people will take part, what tests they will receive, and how treatment will progress.

Every protocol must be approved by the organization sponsoring the study and also by the Institutional Review Board of each hospital or study site taking part. The purpose of this approval process is to protect you.

Meeting eligibility guidelines

All participants in a clinical trial must meet eligibility guidelines. Some of these guidelines may include

- Age
- Gender
- Type of cancer
- Stage of cancer
- Treatment history
- General health

Including participants who all meet the same eligibility criteria provides a level playing field for the study and helps produce reliable results regarding which patient groups will benefit most from the new treatment. The criteria also serve to exclude any would-be participants who may be harmed in any way by the experimental drugs or treatments that are part of the study.

Knowing your rights

All participants in cancer treatment studies have rights. When you participate in a clinical trial, it's helpful to know these rights, as they are designed to protect you. For example, you have the right to

- ✔ **Make your own decisions:** Don't give in to pressure. Talk with your doctor, talk with the clinical trial staff, and talk with your family, but make the decision yourself.

- ✔ **Expect to be monitored:** If you do decide to participate, the clinical trial staff must monitor your response to treatment throughout the study.

- ✔ **Expect to be safe:** If a treatment harms you in any way, you will be removed from the study and may seek other treatment from your own doctor.

- ✔ **Leave if you want to:** You have the right to leave any study at any time.

Some people think that if you sign on the dotted line to take part in a clinical trial you must stay in the study no matter what. That's not true. The document that you sign before beginning a clinical trial is a consent form. This document represents your right to informed consent. That means you must be presented with all the facts in writing about the study before you decide whether to take part. The document typically contains details about the treatments, the tests, the benefits, and risks of the study. During the study, you may be informed of new findings, such as new side effects or new risks. Once again, you may be asked to sign a document saying you have been informed of these new side effects and new risks and that you choose to stay. If you don't choose to stay, of course, you are free to go.

Feeling Good About Taking Part

If you do decide to take part and go the distance in the clinical trial, well — good for you! Cancer clinical trials have served to advance cancer prevention, treatment, and diagnosis enormously, and that's in spite of the fact that less than 5 percent of all adults diagnosed with cancer each year — some 40,000 to 45,000 people — take part in clinical trials. Among children with cancer, more than 75 percent participate in clinical trials. Many researchers think that the difference between the percentage of adults who participate in clinical trials and the percentage of children who participate has resulted in the fact that more children are cured of their cancers than adults.

Why do such a small percentage of adults participate?

Exploring why more doctors don't conduct trials

In the July 19, 2004, edition of *American Medical News,* a publication of the American Medical Association, reporter Damon Adams writes that according to a poll by Harris Interactive, Inc., 11 percent of the 431 physicians surveyed were "interested in becoming clinical investigators but did not know where to get started" while 17 percent "were not interested" in such work. The poll, conducted in May of 2004, also found that "only 13 percent of practicing physicians were serving as clinical investigators," and fully half of the doctors who responded had never conducted a clinical trial.

Among the reasons the doctors listed for not conducting a clinical trial were

✔ No opportunity to do so

✔ Time commitment is too much

✔ Not enough personnel support

✔ Not enough resources

✔ Burdensome paperwork

Many people are unaware of the existence of these scientific studies because many doctors don't take the time to inform or enroll patients. Often, the doctors simply do not have the staff or funding to do so. This is unfortunate for two important reasons. First, doctors and researchers already know that improvements in cancer are a direct result of clinical trials. Second, an increasing number of anticancer drugs are being developed, and more physicians are needed to help test them.

Hearing what participants have to say

Surveys about clinical trials show that more people are becoming aware that they exist. For example, in 2004, Harris Interactive, Inc., surveyed 5,822 adults, 656 of whom had participated in clinical trials exploring treatments for a number of diseases. Harris had taken similar surveys in previous years, and between 2001 and 2004 the number of people who said they had the opportunity to participate in clinical trials jumped from 13 percent to 19 percent. The actual number of participants in clinical trials also grew modestly, from 8 percent in 2001 to 11 percent in 2004.

The people polled listed numerous reasons for participating in a clinical trial, including the following:

✔ To advance medicine or science

✔ To earn extra money

- ✔ To help others with the same medical condition
- ✔ To obtain better treatment
- ✔ To obtain education for the treatment of their disease
- ✔ To improve their health

Most of the respondents reported that participating was a positive experience, and few said they had had any second thoughts. That said, about half the people polled in 2004 said they believe that those who participate in clinical trials are "like guinea pigs" and that they are "taking a gamble with their health."

Banishing the notion of guinea pigs

This guinea pig business is nothing new. In 2000, Harris Interactive, Inc., conducted a survey of nearly 6,000 people diagnosed with cancer. Eight out of 10 patients surveyed said they were unaware that clinical trials could be an option for them. Among those patients who knew about clinical trials, 71 percent said they had chosen not to participate. Fears expressed by the respondents included

- ✔ Receiving a placebo in place of actual treatment
- ✔ Getting treatment inferior to standard methods
- ✔ Being treated like a "guinea pig"

Now let's hear from those who did participate.

The majority of people polled who had participated in clinical trials rated their experience as positive. According to the report, "Ninety-seven percent said they were treated with dignity and respect, and received excellent or good quality care. Some 81 percent said they were not subjected to more tests and procedures than they thought necessary. And 82 percent said they were not treated like 'guinea pigs.'"

Most importantly, three out of four said they would recommend participation in a clinical trial to someone else with cancer. With that in mind, if you have chosen to participate in a clinical trial, give yourself a pat on the back.

Chapter 7

Getting a Second Chance: Bone Marrow Transplants

Make no mistake: A bone marrow transplant is serious business. If your doctor has recommended this procedure, it's because it's time to bring out the really big guns — a phrase that gives the nod to the vocabulary of war used so often in discussions of cancer treatments. To continue the metaphor, if you think of fighting cancer as fighting the enemy within, a bone marrow transplant is a major assault.

Mounting a major assault, one that goes beyond chemotherapy and radiation therapy, is scary. Your hospital stay may be lengthy, maybe three weeks or more. You likely will become very ill during the treatments just prior to the bone marrow transplant. The procedure itself can cause unpleasant side effects. The first 24 hours after the transplant can be physically difficult. A host of precautions must be taken during the time that your immune system works to rebuild. And full recovery may take a year or more.

The best defense is to arm yourself with information as you proceed. Also, you would do well to remember that people who have had the procedure and now live normal, healthy lives sometimes refer to a bone marrow transplant as a miracle.

Surely, there is magic in this procedure, but it is magic based on medical science. In this chapter, you gain a better understanding of what a bone marrow transplant is, how it works, how to prepare yourself for the procedure, and what to expect during the recovery process.

Demystifying Bone Marrow Transplants

A bone marrow or stem cell transplant — a Herculean effort to rebuild a damaged or weakened system — is commonly used to treat these forms of cancer:

- Leukemia
- Lymphoma
- Multiple myeloma
- Childhood brain tumors and certain inherited deficiencies of the immune system
- *Neuroblastoma,* an uncommon cancer known to occur most often in children

More than 15,000 bone marrow transplants are performed in the United States every year, and this treatment is ever evolving. Clinical trials are underway to study the value of bone marrow transplants in treating other types of cancer.

Defining bone marrow

Bone marrow transplants are a complex subject, so we'll take first things first.

What is bone marrow?

Bone marrow is a soft, spongelike material found in the central cavity of bones. The marrow contains immature cells called *stem cells* that produce blood cells. When you're born, you have active marrow in every bone, and blood cell development is at the height of its production. By the time you're a young adult, the marrow in your hands, feet, arms, and legs has taken early retirement and stopped producing blood cells. Bones that keep up the work of blood cell development throughout the rest of your life include the backbones (vertebrae), hip bones, shoulder bones, ribs, breastbone, and skull.

Most stem cells are in the bone marrow, but some circulate through the blood. Through a process called *hematopoiesis,* the stem cells produce white blood cells (leukocytes) to fight infection, red blood cells (erythrocytes) to carry oxygen through the body, and platelets (thrombocytes), which are clotting agents — see Figure 7-1. You need both types of blood cells and platelets to keep your immune system healthy. The smallest infection could wreak havoc in your body without these important components.

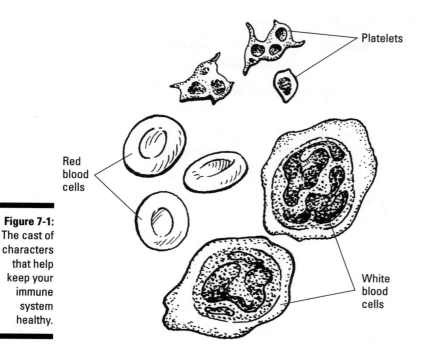

Platelets

Red blood cells

White blood cells

Identifying the purpose of a transplant

Originally, bone marrow or stem cell transplants were used as a last resort for treating leukemia. Today, the procedure is used to treat a number of illnesses, often earlier in the course of the disease than in the past. If you have one of the types of cancer commonly treated with a transplant, if your cancer is not responding to standard treatment, or if cancer previously treated has come back, undergoing a bone marrow or stem cell transplant gives you a second chance.

The transplant process involves *conditioning,* or treatment with very high doses of chemotherapy and/or radiation therapy. In Chapters 4 and 5, we explain how chemotherapy and radiation therapy work. In short, chemotherapy and radiation therapy kill cells that divide rapidly — a definition that fits cancer cells and also bone marrow cells. You need healthy bone marrow stem cells in order to make the blood cells that carry oxygen, protect you from infection, and prevent bleeding. The purpose of heavy doses of chemotherapy and radiation prior to a bone marrow transplant is threefold:

- ✔ To eliminate diseased bone marrow
- ✔ To reduce the number of cancer cells in the body
- ✔ To suppress the immune system to prevent rejection of the transplant

During the bone marrow or stem cell transplant, healthy stem cells are transplanted to replace those destroyed by the large doses of chemotherapy and radiation therapy. The goal, then, is that over time the transplanted stem cells will work to restore the bone marrow's ability to produce the blood cells you need, and a healthy production schedule will be resumed.

Recognizing the source of stem cells

Stem cells needed for bone marrow transplants come from three sources:

- ✔ Bone marrow
- ✔ Peripheral blood
- ✔ Umbilical cord

The stem cells may be your own, or they may come from a donor. Collecting stem cells from either the patient's or a donor's bone marrow is the traditional method used, and it's performed in an operating room. (More about that in a minute.) When stem cells are taken from the blood, surgery is not required. Instead, the retrieval procedure is much like donating blood. These stem cells are called *peripheral blood stem cells*. Stem cells also can be collected from cord blood that remains in the placenta and the umbilical cord of a newborn baby. Umbilical cord stem cells are harvested, frozen, and stored for future use after the baby's birth. This procedure must be arranged several months before the delivery.

Exploring the Types of Transplants

Three types of bone marrow transplants are performed:

- ✔ **Autologous transplants,** in which you receive your own stem cells
- ✔ **Syngeneic transplants,** in which you receive stem cells from an identical twin
- ✔ **Allogeneic transplants,** in which you receive stem cells from a relative or an unrelated donor

All three types of transplants are complicated, expensive procedures, and bone marrow transplants cannot be performed just anywhere. More than 150 transplant centers affiliated with the National Marrow Donor Program are scattered across the country. If you live near a center, you're set. If you don't, or if the center near you is small and has performed few transplants, you need to locate a center farther from your home. For a state-by-state list of centers affiliated with the National Marrow Donor Program, call 888-999-6743, or visit www.marrow.org and click on Patient Resources.

Typically, a bone marrow transplant requires a prolonged hospital stay, all of it spent in isolation in a single room. A bone marrow transplant may cost from $50,000 to $250,000, depending on the type of transplant. If you have health insurance coverage, many of the costs of the procedure, the recovery period, and the follow-up care likely will be covered. If you do not have health insurance, some charitable agencies, service organizations, and government programs make funds available. The Cancer Information Service at the National Cancer Institute has information about sources of financial assistance; you can call 800-422-6237 or visit www.cancer.gov for information. Or you may want to speak with a social worker on staff at your transplant treatment center for more information on available financial resources.

If you need an allogeneic transplant, friends and co-workers may offer to be tested as potential donors. A simple blood test, performed perhaps at a local Red Cross office, gets the process started. Not everybody is eligible to donate bone marrow. For instance, anyone with a history of heart disease, cancer, hepatitis, insulin-dependent diabetes, or HIV is not eligible. The Red Cross, of course, screens all potential donors. But in this situation, you don't have to count on just your immediate circle of friends.

Several international organizations maintain registries to help find matches for people who need a bone marrow transplant from a nonrelative. See the "Searching for a Donor" section, later in the chapter, for more information.

Your doctor will recommend which type of transplant would work best for you. In the following sections, we take a closer look at each.

Looking at autologous transplants

Technically, an autologous transplant is actually a transfer of bone marrow cells out of you and then back in. First, the cells are *harvested,* or retrieved. Then they are cleaned, or purged, of any lingering cancer cells to minimize the chance of cancer coming back. Sometimes, purging damages some healthy marrow cells, so the doctor may need to obtain additional marrow before the transplant. Next, the bone marrow cells are treated with a protective agent that allows them to be frozen without being damaged until it's time for them to be thawed and returned to your body.

The advantage of autologous transplants, of course, is that the body has no reason to reject its own marrow or blood stem cells. In the other two types of transplants, doctors must work to ensure that the transplanted marrow matches the patient's own marrow as closely as possible. The way to do that is through a special blood test that identifies an individual's set of proteins, called *human leukocyte-associated (HLA) antigens,* on the surface of the cells. The closer the match between your sets of proteins and those of the donor, the more likely the transplantation will be successful and the complications minimal.

Looking at syngeneic transplants

Syngeneic transplantation is rare because identical twins also are rare. However, because identical twins have the same genes, they also have identical sets of HLA antigens. That means identical twins make ideal donors for one another.

Looking at allogeneic transplants

Again, the success of all transplantation depends on how well the HLA antigens of the donor's marrow match those of the recipient's marrow. The higher the number of matching HLA antigens, the greater the chance that your body will accept the donor's bone marrow. You may think that anyone with brothers or sisters would find a likely match. However, only 30 to 40 percent of transplantation patients have a sibling or parent with the six HLA matches required for a successful outcome.

In recent years, there has been an increase in the use of marrow from unrelated donors, though the chances of obtaining HLA-matched marrow from an unrelated donor are small. Again, there's that necessary match of six key antigens.

Looking at an alternative

An emerging alternative to a traditional allogeneic transplant is the *minitransplant.* Currently, the minitransplant is available only in clinical trials.

Researchers are studying its use as a treatment for leukemia, lymphoma, multiple myeloma, melanoma, and kidney cancer.

A key difference between a traditional allogeneic transplant and a minitransplant is the preparation process. A minitransplant uses lower, less toxic doses of chemotherapy and/or total body irradiation (radiation therapy to the entire body) prior to an allogeneic transplant. This treatment eliminates some, but not all, of the bone marrow. As with traditional pretransplant treatment, a minitransplant treatment reduces the number of cancer cells and suppresses the immune system to help prevent rejection of the transplant.

Another difference with the minitransplant is that your bone marrow cells and cells from the donor may coexist in your body afterward. When the donor's bone marrow cells begin to produce new white blood cells, red blood cells, and platelets, they may cause what is called a *graft-versus-tumor effect* and may work to destroy the cancer cells that were not eliminated by the anticancer drugs and/or total body irradiation. To boost this desirable effect, you may be given an injection of the donor's white blood cells. This procedure is called a *donor lymphocyte infusion*.

Searching for a Donor

As we note earlier in the chapter, several organizations maintain registries to help find matches for people who need a bone marrow transplant from a non-relative. One of the largest such groups in the United States is the National Marrow Donor Program, a federally funded, nonprofit organization based in Minneapolis. You can visit www.marrow.org or call 800-627-7692 for more information about this organization. The National Marrow Donor Program maintains an international registry of volunteer potential donors for all sources of blood stem cells used in transplantation.

Don't think that you have to sit down at the computer, find a registry, and plead your case. Your doctor will recommend a transplant center qualified to perform a transplant, and the staff at that center will begin a preliminary donor search for you for free.

These searches take time, especially if a preliminary search doesn't turn up any matches for you. Additional donors are added to the registries on a regular basis, so don't give up. If matches are available, then a formal search is in order to consider each candidate more carefully. A formal search may involve a fee, and you'll also want to check with your insurance company about what expenses are covered. Typically, would-be donors pay only for a screening test to join the national registry. Recipients — or their insurance companies — pay for the formal donor search, retrieval costs, and any transportation costs for the frozen bone marrow.

Preparing for a Bone Marrow Transplant

No question about it, preparing yourself emotionally for a bone marrow transplant is trying. In fact, it's quite a bit like the emotional roller coaster ride you took when you first learned that you had cancer. You're likely to be scared, despondent, and even angry part of the time. After all, you've already gone through a lot with the cancer diagnosis — and now this. However, you may also spend part of the time filled with optimism over the opportunity for a second chance.

Acknowledging your emotions

You definitely won't help yourself if you try to suppress your emotional response to the news that you need a bone marrow transplant. Acknowledge your feelings. Ask for the emotional support you need from family, friends, and co-workers, and get professional help if you're so inclined. You may even want to speak with a trained peer volunteer who has had a bone marrow transplant. The National Bone Marrow Transplant Link (800-546-5268 or www.nbmtlink.org) can help you find such a person, as can the Leukemia & Lymphoma Society (800-955-4572 or www.leukemia-lymphoma.org).

Learning from Lot's wife

In her book *Do As I Say, Not As I Did* (Perigee Books), author Wendy Reid Crisp has this to say about second chances:

"We want a second chance, on our own terms, on our own schedules. Opportunity doesn't work that way: if an angel grabs you by the hand and pulls you out of an exploding city, get a move on. We know why Mrs. Lot turned around: she missed her neighbors; in the rush, she'd forgotten her favorite pots; she wanted a final good-bye. Lot's wife was changed into a pillar of salt, and we will be, too, from the salt of our own tears. 'I should never have left L.A. What would that stock in Disney be worth today? I wish I'd taken that job. Why wasn't I a better mother? Where did the money go?'

"A second chance, or a third, or a fourth, requires a complete commitment: head into a new land unburdened by disappointments, empowered by experience, and eyes forward."

You don't have to do this alone. And you do want to try to do it your own way. Ask the staff at your transplant center if you may bring in headphones and a small CD player so that you may listen to soothing music or meditation tapes in the days leading up to the transplant and perhaps during the process itself. Another way to personalize the experience is to bring one or two photos of family members or friends for your room. You may even be permitted to bring a favorite plush stuffed toy to serve as a good luck charm. Do ask about these possibilities and any other personal touches that would help comfort you.

Appointing a caregiver

Not only do you not *have* to go through this experience alone, you *can't* do it alone. Someone — or several someones, which will make it easier on everyone — needs to be available to carry out a number of important tasks as you prepare for the bone marrow transplant, undergo the procedure, and begin the recovery process. There is much to do. A spouse, relative, or friend who likely shares your anxiety about the transplant may welcome an opportunity to serve as the caregiver, but all things considered, this is a job best shared by two or three people so that a single caregiver doesn't end up in need of care for him or herself.

The responsibilities of your caregivers include

- ✔ Providing emotional support
- ✔ Providing physical care during and after the transplant
- ✔ Keeping records of medication given
- ✔ Reporting unusual symptoms to the healthcare team
- ✔ Informing relatives and friends of your condition
- ✔ Preparing a safe, welcoming environment at home for you
- ✔ Driving you to and from the hospital for follow-up care
- ✔ Helping you practice self-care

With the help of your caregivers, make whatever plans you need to make that will best help you get through the coming months. Call on your coping skills that helped to get you through the cancer diagnosis. Educate yourself about the bone marrow transplant procedure and the recovery period so you know exactly what to expect. And take time to remind yourself that, as with other challenges in life, you have to move straight through this experience — no matter how difficult it is — in order to come out smiling on the other side.

Comparing Retrieval Methods

Maybe you are providing your own bone marrow/stem cells for the transplant (that's an autologous transplant), or maybe you have found a donor (that's a syngeneic transplant if from an identical twin or an allogeneic transplant if from anyone else). Either way, the method of retrieving the bone marrow is the same. To avoid confusion, we speak of the *donor* here even if that happens to be you.

Harvesting the bone marrow

Typically, the donor is placed under general anesthesia in an operating room. Then, the doctor makes several tiny cuts in the skin on the back above the hip bone. Next, he inserts a large needle through the cuts directly into the bone marrow, which is drawn out through the needle. The procedure takes about an hour and results in a "harvest" of about 5 to 10 percent of the donor's bone marrow.

In a laboratory, technicians process the bone marrow to remove blood and any bone fragments. Next, the bone marrow is combined with a preservative and placed in a liquid nitrogen freezer to keep the stem cells alive until they're needed for transplantation. This technique is called *cryopreservation*.

Though the donor's back may be a bit sore for a few days or the donor may feel tired, the bone marrow retrieval process rarely causes any significant health problems for the donor. Over the next few weeks, the donor's body will replace the amount of marrow donated.

Obtaining peripheral blood stem cells

Peripheral blood stem cells are retrieved through a process called *apheresis* or *leukapheresis*. The number of stem cells in the blood is much lower than the number found in bone marrow. To boost the number of stem cells in the blood before retrieval, the donor may be asked to take a medication known as *colony stimulating factor* or *growth factor* for four or five days before apheresis. When the medication has kicked in and the number of stem cells released into the bloodstream has increased, apheresis can take place.

No anesthesia is required for apheresis. In this procedure, a technician removes blood either through a *central venous catheter,* which is a flexible tube placed in a large vein in the neck or chest, or through a needle placed in a large vein in the donor's arm. The blood cycles through a machine that removes the stem cells, and then the blood is returned to the donor. The stem cells collected may be treated with chemotherapy drugs to destroy any cancer cells that may be present, and then the stem cells are frozen until they're needed for transplantation.

Apheresis can take four to six hours. Usually, the donor feels no pain, though there may be some discomfort. For instance, the donor may feel lightheaded or have chills. Some people experience numbness around the lips or cramping in the hands. The colony stimulating factor given prior to the procedure sometimes causes bone and muscle aches or headaches, or the donor may have difficulty sleeping. Generally, all the side effects stop within two to three days after the last dose of the medication.

Undergoing the Rescue Process

The transfer of the bone marrow or the peripheral blood stem cells is called the *rescue process*. Again, this process is hard. The preparation is hard, the procedure is hard, and the recovery period is hard. Still, hope is part of the entire process when you think of it as a rescue.

Experiencing external changes

You receive the transplanted products through a *central venous catheter*, a flexible tube placed in a large vein in the neck or chest. But before you can be "rescued," you receive high doses of chemotherapy through the catheter to kill the last of the cancer cells in your body. Typically, this process takes three to seven days, depending on the regimen. Potential side effects may include

- ✔ Nausea
- ✔ Vomiting
- ✔ Fatigue
- ✔ Loss of appetite
- ✔ Mouth sores
- ✔ Hair loss
- ✔ Skin reactions

During the transplant itself, you may experience nausea and vomiting, and sometimes chills and fever hang around for the first 24 hours after the transplant.

Experiencing internal changes

Immediately after the rescue process, you are exceptionally susceptible to infection and bleeding. That said, you will be closely monitored and kept in the hospital for anywhere from 10 to 35 days, depending on your condition.

Many changes will take place internally in the coming months. For instance, after they enter the bloodstream, the transplanted cells travel to the bone marrow. There, in a process known as *engraftment,* the transplanted cells will begin to produce new white blood cells, red blood cells, and platelets. Engraftment kicks in three to four weeks after your rescue. The doctor will monitor the engraftment with frequent blood tests. Other blood tests will show whether your cancer has returned. *Bone marrow aspiration* — a procedure where the doctor removes a small sample of bone marrow through a needle for examination under a microscope — helps your doctor determine how well the new marrow is working.

Even if it's working well, engraftment is only the beginning of the recovery process for your immune system. If you have an autologous transplant, recovery can take several months. If you have an allogeneic or syngeneic transplant, your body may need as long as two years to recover fully.

Keeping an Eye Out for Post-Rescue Problems

In the first weeks of recovery, a number of health problems can develop. Among them are

- **Bacterial infections:** Because your immune system is so severely depressed after a bone marrow transplant, you are more susceptible to bacterial infections. Make no mistake: Your temperature will be carefully monitored, and if a fever spikes, you will be treated immediately with antibiotics.

- **Graft-versus-host disease:** Another possible complication after an allogeneic bone marrow transplant is a condition known as *graft-versus-host disease,* which sometimes develops when white blood cells from the donor marrow (the graft) identify the cells of the patient's body (the host) as foreign and attack it. About one-third to one-half of allogeneic transplant recipients develop this disease, which may manifest as a minor skin rash, a disruption in liver function, or gastrointestinal distress. Most cases are mild, and long-term effects are rare. Of course, your doctor will be on the lookout for any signs of the disease, which is treated with steroids or another immunosuppressive agent. Clinical trials are underway to find ways to prevent graft-versus-host disease.

✔ **Bleeding:** Because your supply of platelets is low after a transplant, you are at risk for bleeding. (Platelets allow blood to clot.) You may experience nosebleeds, bleeding gums, or bruising. If your platelet count drops too low, you may need a transfusion of platelets. You may also need a transfusion of red blood cells.

✔ **Pneumonia:** Interstitial pneumonia — a nonbacterial, nonfungal form of pneumonia that penetrates the area between the cells in the lungs — is another potential complication. Again, you will be monitored for signs of pneumonia.

✔ **Graft failure:** This complication takes place when the body cannot accept the new bone marrow (the graft). Symptoms include infection, anemia, and bleeding. Graft failure occurs in only 5 to 15 percent of cases and does not rule out a second transplant.

A bone marrow transplant does carry the potential for some long-term risks, among them:

✔ Infertility

✔ Cataracts

✔ New cancers

✔ Complications in the liver, kidneys, lungs, and/or heart

By all means, talk with your doctor about the likelihood of complications and what to expect after a bone marrow transplant. If this is the procedure that represents a second chance for you, we wish you all the best.

Part III

Chemotherapy: What to Expect and How to Deal with Side Effects

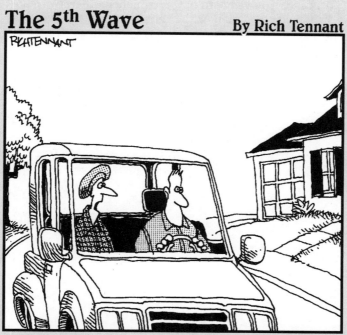

The 5th Wave   By Rich Tennant

"Why didn't you tell me you had the heated seats on? I thought I was having another side effect from the chemo."

In this part . . .

Maybe you've heard how rough chemotherapy treatments are and how the side effects wear you down. This part takes an unblinking look at anticancer drugs and tells you in detail what side effects to expect and how to best deal with them.

Chapter 8

What to Expect During Chemotherapy: A Head-to-Toe Mouthwash

Chemotherapy, a catchall word used for more than 50 different anticancer drugs, has been described in many ways — some of them complimentary and some of them not. Some people refer to chemotherapy drugs as poison, while others think of chemotherapy as a lifesaving potion. Perhaps one of the best descriptions we've heard for chemotherapy is a "head-to-toe mouthwash."

As we explain in Chapter 4, chemotherapy is a systemic treatment that moves through the bloodstream to all parts of the body. We like the mouthwash analogy because of the image it provokes of anticancer drugs moving freely through the body, discovering and killing cancer cells in every nook and cranny from the top of your head to the tip of each toe.

However you choose to think about chemotherapy — and we hope you embrace your treatment, as it may save your life — the job that chemotherapy sets out to do is to cure or control cancer.

In this chapter, you find out what to expect from chemotherapy at your first appointment, and you get some suggestions on how to help make successive treatments go well.

Your First Appointment: Getting the Toughest One Out of the Way

You wake up one morning and realize that this day will be different than all others that have come before, because this is the day you begin chemotherapy treatments. So much has happened in the short period of time that has brought you to this day. A physical symptom or the result of a blood test raised a warning flag. You were tested further and diagnosed with cancer. Perhaps you've had surgery, or maybe you've undergone radiation therapy to shrink a tumor in preparation for surgery or chemotherapy.

You and your doctor have discussed any options you may have regarding your treatment. Together, you have made the best choice, and you have educated yourself about what to expect from the particular regimen. You have discussed what side effects you may experience and put strategies in place to combat them. (For more on side effects from chemotherapy, see Chapters 9, 10, and 11.) You know how many chemotherapy treatments you are to have and when they will take place. As we explain in Chapter 4, chemotherapy treatments generally are scheduled in cycles, most often every two or three weeks, with time in between for your body to recover. How many treatments you need depends on several factors, including the following:

- The kind of cancer
- The type of drugs used
- Your age
- Your general health
- Your body's response to the drugs

The last factor, of course, will be monitored. If you do well, your series of chemotherapy treatments will take place one after another, following logically from the first to the last. However, if chemotherapy is particularly tough for you, your doctor may delay a treatment or two, try a different drug or combination of drugs, or perhaps halt chemotherapy altogether. But that's an issue for another day; you need to focus on right now. For the moment, with your doctor you have mapped out a schedule for the next several months and written the dates on your calendar.

And now here it is: the day you will have your first chemotherapy treatment.

Assessing your feelings

How are you supposed to feel about starting chemotherapy?

How you are *supposed* to feel, of course, doesn't really matter. How you *do* feel is what counts. You may feel anxious or even scared. That's normal. You may feel eager to get started, to get the first one out of the way, so you can find out for yourself what it's like. Then you can mark that first one off the calendar and even start to look forward to future treatments so that eventually, even if it's several months away, you will wake up one day and realize that you've reached the day of your very last chemotherapy treatment.

But we get ahead of ourselves.

Preparing for your first treatment

What will chemotherapy be like for you? Because everyone responds to cancer treatments differently, we can't answer this question precisely. What we can tell you is what that first dose of chemotherapy is like for most people. We also can tell you that typically, a treatment takes about three hours (although you may need a few minutes to get settled ahead of time and a few more to say your goodbyes before you leave).

As we note in Chapter 4, there are three main delivery systems for anticancer drugs and four lesser-used methods. The three main delivery systems are

- Intravenous drip
- Injection
- Pills

Of these three, most people have chemotherapy through the intravenous (IV) drip. In preparation for treatment, many people choose to have a catheter inserted in the chest to make the chemotherapy infusion go more smoothly. We describe the catheter in detail in Chapter 4.

Okay — you've signed up to receive your anticancer drugs through an IV drip, and your catheter has been in place long enough for any resulting swelling to go down. Now do you get in your car and drive to your first chemotherapy treatment?

Not quite yet. You have some tasks to do before you leave for the doctor's office or the medical center.

Filling your prescriptions

Most likely, your doctor or chemo nurse has given you a prescription for anti-nausea medication. You may also have prescriptions for an anti-diarrheal drug and a drug to lessen anxiety. You want to get these prescriptions filled in advance and bring them to your first treatment. There, your chemo nurse will talk with you about these medications and answer any questions you may have.

Eating breakfast or lunch

You want to eat a light meal on the first day of chemotherapy — either breakfast or lunch, depending on what time your appointment begins. This is not the day to indulge in fried or greasy foods. Think protein, and eat something easy to digest.

Don't show up with an empty stomach because that may make you more uncomfortable than if you have a light meal. Doctors recommend that many drugs be taken with food to avoid nausea, and that recommendation applies to anticancer drugs as well.

Getting dressed

Having chemotherapy, we are pleased to report, is not a formal affair. Wear loose, comfortable clothing, and consider dressing in layers. That way, if you become warm, you may shed your sweater or sweatshirt. If you become cold, you have that top layer to put back on. Or you may bring a warm couch throw or afghan to snuggle under.

Confirming your ride

You want to have someone lined up ahead of time to drive you to chemotherapy. Some treatment centers offer plenty of room for your family member or friend to sit with you. At others, your companion may have to wait elsewhere until your treatment is finished. Either way, be certain that you have a ride.

Please don't think that after chemotherapy you will be so incapacitated that you would be unable to drive. That's not the issue here. You may be slightly dizzy or slightly queasy. Or, if you take the anti-nausea medicine before leaving the doctor's office or treatment center (which we discuss in a minute), you may become sleepy. Besides, it's a good idea to have someone along so you can turn to that person and say, "That wasn't so bad."

Arriving for your treatment

As we mention in Chapter 4, some people are admitted to the hospital for chemotherapy treatments, but most people have chemo at the doctor's office, at a clinic, or in a hospital's outpatient department. That's all settled in advance of course, depending on the following:

- ✔ Your insurance company's rules
- ✔ Your doctor's preference
- ✔ Your preference
- ✔ Your chemotherapy drugs

For most people, intravenous chemotherapy is a group experience at an infusion center. Expect to undergo that experience in a sun-filled room with large, overstuffed lounge chairs arranged along the wall — or somewhere equally pleasant. More likely than not, you will have toured the infusion center (or *treatment lounge,* as some people call it) before your first appointment. You also probably have met the chemo nurses and the staff. You can be sure that they will welcome you warmly at your first appointment. Everyone understands that you are jittery about this new experience, so you won't have to explain that. Of course, if you have questions that have come up since your last appointment with your medical oncologist, feel free to ask them.

Chances are that you will have a short meeting with your oncologist before your treatment begins. Then you will be encouraged to choose a cozy lounge chair and settle in.

Undergoing your first treatment

Chemotherapy drugs administered through an IV drip come in large, plastic bags kept in a refrigerated unit. Your chemo nurse will gather up the bags selected for your treatment and hang them on a traditional IV pole next to your chair. One or two of the bags will contain the anticancer drug or drugs prescribed for you. There likely will be a bag of anti-nausea medication that you will receive through the IV (although you may be given anti-nausea pills instead), and you also may notice a bag of *saline solution* — a combination of salt and distilled water. After the nurse has inserted the IV needle into your arm or into the port of your catheter, the combination of medications and the saline solution drips slowly out of the bags and into your bloodstream.

That's all there is to it. You will sit calmly and quietly while you receive your chemotherapy. Some people feel chilled during part of the treatment; if you get cold, ask for a blanket. Some people feel slightly queasy; if you do, speak up. If you are thirsty, ask for a drink of water. Some people feel perfectly normal and begin to wonder what the fuss was all about. They talk quietly with their companion, read, or doze.

Generally, everyone is asked to leave cellphones or computers at home or in the car. Using these devices in the chemotherapy treatment area may interfere with monitoring equipment, possibly endangering the safety of other patients.

Heading for home

At some lovely point in the day, the chemo nurse will tell you that you are finished and unhook you from the IV. Because you have been taking in a lot of fluids, you may wish to use the restroom. Your chemo nurse or a staff member will make sure you know when your next appointment is scheduled. (You should already know, because your schedule will have been set up at a previous appointment.)

You may be asked to schedule a blood test called a *nadir check* in 10 to 14 days to determine your blood count; at that same appointment, you can talk about any side effects you may be experiencing. If you need a lab slip for the test, you will receive it.

Clarifying when to take anti-nausea medication

Horror stories abound about people who routinely experience violent nausea and vomiting after chemotherapy. What you rarely hear are the stories about all the people who never experience any nausea or vomiting at all after chemotherapy. Your doctor or nurse may instruct you to take anti-nausea pills if and when you become queasy. We suggest a more defensive approach.

We know a chemotherapy nurse who routinely reminds her patients that if you wait too long to take that pill, you may not be able to keep it down. This nurse, an angel in disguise, strongly recommends taking an anti-nausea pill with a small cup of water before you leave the treatment center and continuing to take the pills as prescribed for the next 48 hours.

Heeding her advice guarantees that you will be sleepy, a little dizzy, and not (as they say) the sharpest tool in the shed for that 48-hour period. However, you also most likely will experience no nausea and vomiting. It's your call.

Saying goodbye until next time

So you've met some new comrades in arms, as it were, in your battle against cancer. You've not only watched as other people sat calmly having a chemo treatment, you've spoken with some of them, maybe shared a few details of your battle, and asked for a few tips from those more experienced at this routine. You will look for these same faces next time, and you're likely to see some of them. You won't exactly be an "old hand" at chemotherapy by then, but you already know so much more than you did before you walked in the door.

The next thing you know, you've said your goodbyes, and you're getting in the car to head home, where you will eat a meal, take a nap, or maybe call a friend to report on your day. Don't forget to ask that friend to pass along your news to others so you don't spend long, tiring hours on the telephone. Maybe you're even going back to the office, though we can't say we recommend that. Many people are able to work full-time during chemotherapy treatments, making just a few adjustments in their regular schedules. However, your first treatment is bound to be an emotionally tiring experience, and you may feel dizzy or sleepy, so work may not be the best place to go.

None of the side effects of chemotherapy (which we describe in detail in Chapters 9, 10, and 11) set in immediately, so just take it easy after that first treatment.

Continuing with Chemo

You may be wondering if each successive chemotherapy treatment will be identical to the first. In some ways, chemotherapy is a routine: Your chemotherapy treatments are scheduled at intervals that allow the drugs to systematically kill cancer cells that may be in your body at various stages of growth. In other ways, "routine" isn't the right word. For instance, some side effects may occur after one treatment and then never come back. Other side effects may show up after each treatment, sometimes staying the same and sometimes growing in intensity. We can't tell you exactly what will happen to you — we simply don't know. Everyone responds to cancer therapies differently. Only time will tell.

That said, we have some suggestions that we think will help make your chemotherapy treatments go more successfully.

One thing you can do for yourself during chemo is drink water. Bring your own bottle, or bring a glass to fill from the office water cooler. Increased intake of water moves the chemotherapy drugs through your system more readily, not to mention all the other benefits of moisturizing from within.

Keeping your appointments

Your oncologist will explain that to get the best results from anticancer drugs, you need to keep every appointment, showing up for each scheduled treatment for as long as your presence is required. Chemotherapy is a cumulative process — every treatment builds on the last one — so you want to make a point of getting there. However, if an ice storm blows into your city and prevents you from keeping an appointment, don't panic. Call the doctor's office or treatment center and arrange to make up the appointment as soon as possible.

You already have your schedule set up, so you know that appointments generally are available only Monday through Friday. Usually, the doctor's office or treatment center is open between 8 a.m. and 4 p.m. Why the banker's hours? Frankly, the medical profession operates like big business. The employees may wear white coats or blue scrubs, but the specialty "service departments" are fully staffed only during regular business hours so the doctors and nurses have time at night and on weekends to spend with their families too. Still, you can generally schedule treatments at times that suit you. Maybe you've decided to get each treatment out of the way at the beginning of the week, or maybe it works best for your schedule to be on the anti-nausea drugs over the weekend, so you can sleep all you like.

Reporting changes in your health

Your health is closely monitored throughout your chemotherapy treatments. One thing your doctor watches for is a drop in your level of platelets. As we explain in Chapter 7, platelets are blood cells that allow your blood to clot. Sometimes, anticancer drugs affect your bone marrow's ability to make platelets. (In Chapter 9, we talk about special bone marrow stimulants and platelet transfusions that you may need during chemotherapy.)

If you are in between appointments and you notice any bleeding or bruising with no sign of injury, this could be a sign that your blood does not have enough platelets. Call your doctor if any of these symptoms occur:

- Unexpected bruising
- Small, red spots under the skin
- Reddish or pinkish urine
- Black or bloody bowel movements
- Bleeding from the gums or nose

✔ Vaginal bleeding that is new or lasts longer than a regular period

✔ Headaches

✔ Changes in vision

✔ A warm or hot feeling in an arm or leg

Protecting your health

During chemotherapy treatments, you need to take extra precautions to protect your health. Taking these precautions may seem like pampering yourself, and that may not be something that you did often before being diagnosed with cancer. But during treatments, taking precautions is not considered pampering; it's considered good, common sense. Here are some suggestions:

✔ Wash your hands often.

✔ Stay away from people with colds and other contagious illnesses.

✔ Avoid crowds.

✔ Stay away from children who recently have been vaccinated with live viruses.

✔ Avoid cuts or nicks when using scissors, needles, or knives.

✔ Do not get any immunizations without checking with your doctor first.

✔ Wear thick rubber gloves when cleaning up after pets.

✔ Do not eat raw fish, raw seafood, raw meat, or raw eggs.

Here's one more "don't": Don't think for a minute that any unusual side effect or symptom that you experience while undergoing chemotherapy is too trivial to report to your doctor. The whole idea here, the whole point of chemotherapy, is to cure or control your cancer. The method used to do that, by its nature, puts your immune system at risk. Your health is at risk. You are vulnerable. Admit that, be aware of how you can protect yourself, and be vigilant about reporting any fever, injury, or unusual side effects.

Asking for the Support You Need

As you go through cancer treatments, your family and close friends are most likely going to experience a range of emotions. These emotions may include fear, anger, concern, confusion, and helplessness — sometimes all at the same time! If you're the caregiver in your family and the Mother Hen or

Everybody's Rock Solid Guy in your circle of friends, your instinctive response may be to try to comfort the others, assuring them that everything's going to be fine. This is a normal response, but it also may restrict the amount of much-needed emotional support that you receive.

You do everybody concerned a favor when you decide up front to speak openly about how you feel physically — and emotionally — during chemotherapy treatments. When you do so, you are better able to ask for emotional support, as well as for more practical help.

Delegating responsibilities to your family

As you go through chemotherapy, you may decide to provide different levels of information to individual family members about your treatments and side effects, based on their age and health. For instance, knowing all the facts may upset elderly grandparents or young children, so you may want to tell just part of the truth in some cases.

Realizing your spouse's role

Prior to cancer, you and your spouse probably had an established ratio of give-and-take based on years of life experience together. As you quickly discover, cancer changes everything. You may find it helpful — possibly even necessary — for your spouse to take over many of the tasks you're used to doing in your household for the duration of treatment.

While this shift of responsibility may seem like a burden to place on your spouse, that burden likely will be lightly borne because your mate has an opportunity to do something concrete, something specific, something helpful — rather than just sit by your side and fret.

Considering what to ask from your children

Young adults and college-age children likely will appreciate hearing the truth about what you're experiencing. When you deliver that truth, you also can specify what you require in the way of support. "My job right now is to go through chemotherapy," you may say to a son or daughter away at school. "Your job is to get good grades this semester and come home for visits when you can manage it."

Teens still at home can understand the need — and even welcome the opportunity — to pitch in more than before. Even younger children can contribute by playing quietly when Dad or Mom, weary during treatments, needs a nap.

You may want to ask younger children in the family to be in charge of providing you with a good laugh at least twice a day. Children love to tell jokes, and laughter, of course, is good for everybody.

Appointing a "Chemo Buddy"

No matter how involved your immediate family is in caring for you during chemotherapy treatments, all of you will welcome a change of topic — and a change of scene — now and then. Yet sometimes, no matter how eager you are to participate in other conversations or activities that have absolutely nothing to do with cancer, you may find yourself dwelling on your treatments.

Consider asking a close friend — maybe even someone who has been through cancer treatments — to serve as a "Chemo Buddy." Ask this person to promise to listen once a day to all of your thoughts, including your fears, about your treatments. Explain ahead of time that you are looking for someone who will simply listen, sympathize, and wish for a better day for you tomorrow.

Your Chemo Buddy may wish that he could wave a magic wand and return you to your life before cancer, but let that person know that finding someone outside the family willing to listen lends a kind of magic of its own.

Allowing friends to help

Many people — especially women — are eager to help anyone at any time under any circumstances, yet they are reluctant to ask for help themselves. When you're going through chemotherapy treatments, try to remember that receiving is simply the other side of giving. In *The Prophet* (Knopf), the poet and philosopher Kahlil Gibran notes, "You give little when you give of your possessions. It is when you give of yourself that you truly give."

Like many people, most likely you have banked a lot of good deeds in your life, never worrying about payback. Your reward often has been that good feeling you get, a familiar source of quiet pride and contentment, that comes when you know you have made a difference, helped in some way large or small, whether you were recognized for it or not.

Here's a question: No matter how much pride you take in your self-sufficiency, would you deny your friends an opportunity to experience that same delicious good feeling?

Of course not!

Besides, your good friends likely are experiencing the full range of emotions also wreaking havoc with your family's sense of well-being. Frankly, people going through cancer treatments need help, and the people watching you go through treatments need something practical to do to help you in the process. Please give your friends an opportunity to help give you what you need. Kahlil Gibran would be proud.

Hitching rides

When friends ask (and they will) what they can do to help, a terrific answer is to ask for a ride to and from your chemo treatments. As we explain in Chapter 10, one of the common side effects of chemotherapy is fatigue. One big way to lessen that fatigue is to leave the driving to someone else. Asking for a ride is a straightforward, simple request that some of your friends available during the day will be able to fulfill.

If you live a long way from the doctor's office or treatment center, you may feel less guilty about asking for rides if you offer to pay for gas. Your friend may turn that offer down, but asking is a courteous gesture and will emphasize your gratitude for the ride.

Requesting other types of help

If you take time to make a list of specific needs friends can help with, you'll all feel better than if you only express vague notions about what may be helpful. Think about it. In one scenario, a friend asks how to help. You reply that a ride to a treatment would be most appreciated. Your friend asks when to pick you up, you reply, and the two of you have a verbal agreement. You get a ride, and your friend gets to feel good. In another scenario, a friend asks how to help and you reply, "I can't think of anything, but thanks." Your friend may eye you suspiciously but likely will simply say, "Okay, but let me know if anything comes up." You both go away empty-handed.

Specific suggestions on your part as to how friends can help will most likely be met with a smile and a surge of "can do" energy on your friend's part. Of course, your needs during chemotherapy extend beyond transportation.

Here is a list of good deeds you may ask your friends to do for you:

- ✔ Go grocery shopping.
- ✔ Run to the bank.
- ✔ Make a hearty stew or bake a chicken.
- ✔ Pick up stamps at the post office.

- ✔ Bring over a stack of interesting magazines.
- ✔ Make an appointment for a massage for you and drive you there.
- ✔ Get the latest mystery at the library for you.

These all are errands you could easily do before you started chemotherapy. Now, these are just the kinds of side trips that can add to the fatigue caused by the treatments.

Giving Yourself a Break

Of course, there is one thing that only you can do for yourself. You can routinely give yourself a break — cut yourself some slack — and not just in times of true duress. Remember, everything changes when you are diagnosed with cancer. Many of the changes in your routine at home and at work are temporary, in place only for that period of time necessary while going through your treatments. Still, right now you are handling a lot, both physically and emotionally. Peace with these changes comes as you adapt to the new "normal," as you grow to trust your doctors, and as you refine your strategy for success. Along the way, make it easy on yourself. Give yourself a break whenever possible.

Going through chemotherapy asks a lot of a person. It stands to reason that you would allow yourself to get by with doing less than if you were not on anticancer drugs. Instead of bemoaning what you're not getting done, look again at that "to do" list and cross off at least two or three items.

Keeping everything in perspective

Getting through months of chemotherapy successfully takes a keen sense of perspective. You know that your health is the first priority. You know that you must make it to every treatment and take good care of yourself.

Still, as the days turn into weeks and the weeks turn into months and you're still going for chemotherapy, it's not uncommon to get down-hearted. Maybe the idea of all the scary drugs in your system gives you the creeps. Maybe the rash on your head from your wig is getting worse. Maybe you awaken in the middle of the night spooked about your future. Maybe — most likely — you're ready to get all this over with and get on with your life.

A cellular consensus

Your coauthor Patricia met a man in her cancer support group at The Wellness Community in St. Louis who spoke often of good "cellular health" as his priority. He was well aware that his treatments were targeting cancerous cells in his body, and he decided to do what he could to help get healthy at a cellular level as well.

The man held a stressful job that often involved intense, cut-throat bargaining sessions held on the telephone. "A few days ago, I was hollering into the phone, doing my job, and all of a sudden the thought crossed my mind that all this stress, all the shouting, could not possibly be good for my cells," the man told Patricia. He said that he made an excuse to hang up the phone and went for a short walk to cool down. His approach to his job was different after that. He said, "From now on, I'm only doing what's good for my cells."

When fears rise up and you're too tired to battle back with any serious effort, talk with your family, your friends, and your doctors. Reevaluate your success strategies, and consider adding another member to your survival team (see Part V for some suggestions).

Keeping an eye on the future

If you get discouraged and start asking yourself why you are going to all this trouble, showing up every three weeks — just about the time you're starting to feel like yourself again — and filling up with more drugs that you know will bring you down, here's a gentle reminder: You got cancer, and now you're getting it fixed. The process is not as simple as replacing the alternator in your car when it goes out or replacing a bald tire, but the analogy may be helpful to remember. You got cancer. You're getting it fixed. The good news is that being treated for cancer is an experience with a beginning and an end. What's going on now will not be going on later, so carry on!

Chapter 9

Gimme a Boost: Immune and Bone Marrow Stimulants

*Y*ou already know that chemotherapy kills cancer cells. In the process, chemotherapy also interferes with your body's production of white blood cells, red blood cells, and platelets. This interference may cause serious side effects that must be addressed, as these cells play important roles in your immune system.

White blood cells, red blood cells, and platelets all are produced in stem cells in your bone marrow, which is a soft, spongelike material found in the central cavity of bones. Think of your bone marrow as a factory vital to the health of your body. Think of chemotherapy treatments as periodic bombing raids on cancer cells that also cause damage to that vital factory. Your oncologist knows that you need a renewable source of white blood cells, red blood cells, and platelets, and has several strategies to help clean up after the raid and get the factory in production again.

All told, the risks of chemotherapy are extensive. In fact, in this book you find three entire chapters on possible side effects of anticancer drugs: the one you're reading now, plus Chapters 10 and 11. Keep in mind that these adverse effects counterbalance some extremely positive effects of chemotherapy — namely tumor shrinkage, disease-free survival, and overall survival of cancer.

In this chapter, we explain what side effects may occur at the cellular level and what medications and treatments are available to come to the aid of your immune system as you go through chemotherapy. We also give our opinion about taking nutritional supplements that are said to boost the immune system.

Boning Up on Bone Marrow

As we explain in Chapter 7, when you're born, you have active marrow in every bone, with blood cell development at the height of its production. By the time you're a young adult, the marrow in your hands, feet, arms, and legs stops producing blood cells. The backbones (vertebrae), hip bones, shoulder bones, ribs, breastbone, and skull continue to produce marrow throughout the rest of your life. Inside the marrow are immature stem cells, where blood cells get their start. A smaller number of stem cells circulates through the blood.

Through a process called *hematopoiesis,* stem cells produce white blood cells (leukocytes) to fight infection, red blood cells (erythrocytes) to carry oxygen through the body, and platelets (thrombocytes), which are clotting agents. Both types of blood cells and the platelets work to keep your immune system healthy.

Even when you are in good health, some infections can wreak havoc in your body and overcome a fully functioning immune system — just talk to anybody who has had the flu or a prolonged bout with bronchitis. During chemotherapy treatments, when you are taking anticancer drugs to kill or control cancer, the chemotherapy itself wreaks havoc on your bone marrow and, by extension, on your immune system.

Here's what happens: At the same time that chemotherapy acts on the rapidly dividing cancer cells, the anticancer drugs also act on rapidly dividing cells in the bone marrow. Basically, whenever you have a chemotherapy treatment, the production of red blood cells, white blood cells, and platelets is interrupted. As a result, the number of blood cells circulating in the bloodstream is reduced over time. This may lead to one of four side effects:

- *Leukopenia,* a decreased overall white blood cell count
- *Neutropenia* or *granulocytopenia,* a decrease in the component of white blood cells that protects you against bacterial infections
- *Anemia,* a decreased red blood cell count
- *Thrombocytopenia,* a low platelet count

Your doctor can predict when your chemotherapy treatments will cause the blood counts in your body to drop to their lowest point. This point is called the *nadir.* Many anticancer drugs have a nadir of 7 to 14 days. At that time, blood tests will reveal that white blood cells, red blood cells, and platelets all are reduced in your bloodstream. After a few days, the blood counts begin to rise back to normal.

Here's the catch: Within a few days after your blood counts approach normal levels, it is time once again for a chemotherapy treatment, and the whole cycle begins again.

Of course, your doctor will not rely only on her predictive powers. A quick blood test can reveal your blood counts. If the counts are dangerously low, your doctor will take steps to improve the function of the stem cells in your bone marrow and blood.

Boosting the Immune System

Doctors have different strategies to boost the production of white blood cells, red blood cells, and platelets. Colony stimulating factors, also called *growth factors,* are one treatment available to increase production of white blood cells and red blood cells. These substances, which naturally occur in the body in small amounts, have been duplicated in the laboratory in much larger amounts and work to encourage your bone marrow to increase production of the cells you need. Sometimes, a transfusion is called for to help boost your immune system.

The following sections contain specific information on the treatments available.

White blood cells

White blood cells help the body to fight infections. In Chapter 2 we explain that white blood cells often are heroes, racing to the front lines to fend off all sorts of invaders that may cause infections or disease. When you undergo chemotherapy, some of these white blood cells (the neutrophils) are destroyed in short order, which decreases your body's ability to fight off infection. (A low overall white blood cell count is called *leukopenia,* and the words for a reduction in neutrophils are *neutropenia* and *granulocytopenia.*) Reduced levels of these cells represent a serious side effect, but you need not worry how to recognize the symptoms of leukopenia or neutropenia. A blood test will catch the condition long before you do.

Turning to medical intervention

If your doctor determines from a routine blood test after your first chemotherapy treatment that your white blood cell count has dropped fast and far, he may opt to treat you then — and also after successive chemotherapy appointments — with a colony stimulating factor. This treatment can prevent the white blood cell count from dropping quite as far, or it can help the count to recover more quickly.

These drugs are given by injection, often starting a day or two after chemotherapy and possibly continuing every day for a week or more, though sometimes longer-acting colony stimulating factors that require less frequent injections are used. Are there side effects? Sometimes colony stimulating factors cause a dull ache in the bones, and if you're not prepared for that possibility, it can be scary. Itching around the injection site is another common side effect. These side effects stop after the last injection.

Taking preventative measures

Whether or not you need a colony stimulating factor to help increase your white blood cell production, you can also take simple precautions to protect yourself while your immune system is functioning at a decreased level. None of these precautions is tricky or complicated. In fact, practicing many of them makes common sense all the time to help you stay well. That said, these simple actions are especially important while undergoing chemotherapy. Here they are:

- ✔ **Avoid sick people.** These days, many people show up at the office sick when they should have stayed home in bed. If at all possible, don't share the morning paper, the boss's report, or a bag of chips with anyone at work who has a cold or infection. At home, resist snuggling with any member of the family who is ill.

- ✔ **Wash your hands.** Visit the sink often, not just before and after eating or after using the toilet. Use lots of soap and warm water. Lather up good and go to it.

- ✔ **Avoid cuts and bruises.** Germs hang out in cuts, and this is no time to have to do battle with germs. If you do get a cut or a wound, clean the area well with soap and water. If the cut is shallow, consider pouring hydrogen peroxide over it for extra protection and then put on a sterile bandage. If the cut is deep, call your doctor.

If you are a knife-wielding home cook subject to the occasional accidental cut, consider buying a steel mesh kitchen glove or cut-resistant glove to protect yourself. Kitchenware shops and home goods departments in some stores carry the gloves for about $15.

✔ **Stay out of crowds.** Who knows what germs may lurk in the bodies of fans gathered at a football game, shoppers filling up the mall, or enthusiasts flocking to a music concert? We're not saying you can't have any fun. Just have fun with smaller groups of people right now. And if ever there was a time to learn to love shopping online, this is it. Yes, you will have to pay shipping, but consider it the price of safeguarding your health.

✔ **Eat only cooked food.** Raw fish, raw seafood, raw meat, and raw eggs all may serve as a haven for bacteria. When your immune system is functioning normally, you're not likely to be bothered by this bacteria. During chemotherapy, the bacteria in uncooked food could represent a threat to your health.

✔ **Reassign pet cleanup tasks.** Pet waste — from dogs, cats, birds, and reptiles — is another source of bacteria. If you must be the person responsible for cleaning up after a family pet, wear rubber gloves. After the deed is done, wash the gloves. Then, just to be sure, wash your hands.

Red blood cells

Red blood cells carry oxygen from the lungs to tissues and organs throughout the body. Chemotherapy destroys red blood cells, causing anemia, or a low red blood cell count. Unlike white blood cells, which start dying immediately, red blood cells are harder to knock off, so usually it takes longer for anticancer drugs to affect the red blood cell count. Symptoms of anemia may include

✔ Fatigue

✔ Dizziness

✔ Headache

✔ Lightheadedness

✔ Shortness of breath

✔ Chills

✔ Chest pains

If you have any of these symptoms while undergoing chemotherapy, report them to your doctor.

Turning to medical intervention

If a routine blood test after chemotherapy indicates that your red blood cell count has dropped, your doctor may opt to treat you with a colony stimulating factor (also called a *growth factor*). This treatment can bring your red blood cell count back up.

A common colony stimulating factor used to treat anemia is erythropoietin, also known as EPO. Typically, EPO is given by injection up to three times a week until you are no longer anemic. Are there side effects? Sometimes, EPO can cause flu-like symptoms, a rash, or elevated blood pressure. These side effects stop after the last injection.

If your red blood counts are very low, your doctor may recommend a blood transfusion. Sometimes, blood transfusions can be done on an outpatient basis. It takes two to four hours per unit of blood. A blood transfusion generally cures the anemia.

Today, all blood used in transfusions is carefully screened. Still, if you are concerned, talk to your doctor about asking your family to donate blood products earmarked for you in case you need a transfusion. These things take time, so make these arrangements several weeks in advance.

Taking preventative measures

Whether or not you need a colony stimulating factor to help combat anemia and the fatigue that comes with it, you can also take simple precautions to protect yourself while your immune system is functioning at a decreased level. None of these precautions is tricky or complicated. In fact, practicing many of them makes common sense all the time to help stay well. That said, these simple actions are especially important while undergoing chemotherapy. Here they are:

✔ **Get more rest.** Experts have known for some time that most people require eight hours of sleep a night for optimum functioning, but experts also know that most adults in the United States sleep less than that — and even brag about it. Some 60 percent of adults experience sleep problems in the course of the week. Furthermore, the National Sleep Foundation has reported that "a full 45 percent of adults agree that they will sleep less in order to accomplish more." (So much for showing any interest in functioning optimally!)

If ever you are in need of a good night's sleep, night after night, it's when you undergo chemotherapy treatments. So whatever it is you do instead of going to bed at a reasonable hour, stop it and turn in for the night.

✔ **Pace yourself.** The secret to time management is to determine your priorities, including time for work, time for play, and time for rest. Consider making a grid that allots time slots for each. A little of this, a little of that, a nap on the couch with the cat (or whatever else you had planned) all count and probably can be accomplished if you pace yourself each day, each week, even each month.

✔ **Cut back on "shoulds."** Say you've drawn up a list of what you need to get done, a list that includes errands and chores that don't fit on the aforementioned grid. Should you push yourself to accomplish everything on the list? In the old days, before cancer came into your life, this list would have been a snap. Still, that was then. This is now. Either scratch off half the tasks on the list or give them to someone else to do. That, my friend, is what you "should" do.

Platelets

Platelets are the blood cells that permit the clotting of blood. Clotting is what stops bleeding when you are injured. It should come as no surprise by now that chemotherapy also destroys platelets. The death of these blood cells results in *thrombocytopenia,* a low platelet count. A blood test will reveal a drop in platelets, but some symptoms to watch for include

✔ Small hemorrhages, known as *petechiae,* inside the mouth or on the arms or legs

✔ Excessive bleeding from a cut

✔ Bleeding from the gums after eating a meal or brushing your teeth

✔ Nosebleeds

✔ Easy bruising

Turning to medical intervention

If your doctor determines from a routine blood test after a chemotherapy treatment that your platelet count has dropped, she may opt to treat you with a platelet transfusion. This takes place in a hospital, typically on an outpatient basis. The infusion takes about an hour if all goes well — and usually, it does. Having a platelet transfusion is a lot like having a blood transfusion, but the fluid transfused is clear and contains only platelets. The new platelets typically kick in right away.

Though it is seldom used, a colony stimulating factor, or growth factor, also is available to treat a low platelet count. In special circumstances, depending on the depth and duration of your reduction in platelets, your doctor may recommend the colony stimulating factor instead of a transfusion.

Taking preventative measures

Truth be told, there isn't any way to help prevent a drop in your platelet count. You can — and should — try to protect yourself from cuts and wounds in the kitchen or the garden. If you do get cut, apply pressure to the wound and call your doctor.

An additional complication

Tumor lysis syndrome is another cellular side effect of chemotherapy, but one seldom seen. This syndrome occurs most often in people under treatment for high-grade lymphoma or acute leukemia. Here's how the syndrome occurs: When the anticancer drugs destroy the cancer cells, the body breaks down the dead cells, and the chemicals in these cells are released into your blood. The introduction of these new products changes the normal balance of chemicals circulating in your blood. The following chemicals are already circulating in your blood:

- Potassium
- Sodium
- Phosphate
- Bicarbonate
- Calcium
- Urea

When the normal levels of these chemicals rises as the cancer cells break down, the change can upset your heart rhythm and your kidneys. The best defense, as they say in football, is a good offense. If your doctor thinks you may be at risk for tumor lysis syndrome, he may give you extra fluids and electrolytes (remember the elements on the periodic table you learned in seventh grade?) through an IV drip before your chemotherapy treatment. The extra fluids help flush any extra chemicals out of your body. Drugs such as allopurinol (a tablet) and rasburicase (an IV medication) also can help regulate the chemical balance of your blood. Routine blood tests will keep your doctor informed about whether these measures are working.

Recognizing an Infection

If you develop any of the side effects listed in this chapter, you likely will receive the appropriate supplement or treatment and then continue with your scheduled chemotherapy appointments. However, in some cases, successive chemotherapy treatments may have to be delayed if you become seriously ill. Chemotherapy, like radiation therapy, works best as a cumulative process, so it's best to do everything possible to receive your scheduled treatments.

 We cannot overstate this: You must take meticulous care during cancer treatments to stay as healthy as possible. Anticancer drugs lower your immune system and make you exceptionally vulnerable to colds, infections, and other illnesses.

Now may be a good time to review typical signs of infection. As you go through chemotherapy treatments, be alert for these signs and symptoms:

- Fever above 100.4°F (37.8°C)
- Chills
- Frequent cough
- Excessive drainage
- Sore throat
- Breathlessness
- More than three loose stools in a day
- Pain or burning when urinating

If you think you have an infection, call your oncologist so you can be examined and treated right away with antibiotics. In some cases, you may have to enter the hospital and receive antibiotics intravenously. Sometimes, if you are particularly infection-prone, your doctor may decide to prescribe prophylactic antibiotics before an infection occurs in the hope that the drugs will prevent any infection in your system.

Considering Supplements

Dozens of vitamins, minerals, and herbal supplements claim to boost the body's immune system. Some of the claims may have some merit; many of them simply are advertising slogans. (Some supplements or nutritional treatments even claim to prevent or cure cancer.)

Buyer beware! Little scientific evidence exists that indicates any nutritional supplements boost the immune system or have much to do at all with controlling cancer growth or tolerating anticancer therapy.

The National Institutes of Health has a division devoted to studying dietary supplements (see http://dietary-supplements.info.nih.gov), but at this point, the Food and Drug Administration does not regulate any supplements. Unfortunately, the source of some supplements is not always clear, and because there is no industry standard for quality control, what you get in one bottle may be quite different from what you get in the next. Here are some additional reasons to be wary of relying on supplements to boost your immune system during chemotherapy:

✔ Some supplements can make anticancer drugs less effective.

✔ Some supplements may intensify side effects from chemotherapy.

✔ Some supplements in your system can alter results of blood tests.

If you are a fan of supplements and took them before you were diagnosed with cancer, speak with your doctor about what you take. The two of you can discuss whether you should continue with the supplements or stop taking them until your chemotherapy treatments are over.

The day may come when a nutritional supplement has been scientifically proven to boost parts of the immune system that can control cancer cell growth. On that day, doctors will be among those pleased with the news and likely will recommend the supplements. Until then, you may want to save your money.

Chapter 10

Coping with Serious Side Effects of Chemotherapy

● ●

In This Chapter

▶ Preparing yourself for formidable side effects

▶ Watching out for kidney and bladder damage

▶ Saying "no" to nausea and vomiting

▶ Changing your pace to accommodate fatigue

▶ Battling pain and depression

▶ Anticipating fertility problems

▶ Losing your locks and living through it

● ●

Some cures are comforting, like the honey-sweetened lozenges available to stifle a cough and soothe a raspy throat or the warm bath guaranteed to ease aches from arthritis or overexertion. Anticancer drugs, a time-tested method of curing or controlling cancer, do not soothe or envelop you in comforting warmth. Instead, they storm through your body, intent on crushing every cancer cell they encounter, searching high and low for any cancer cells lingering in out-of-the-way places. This medicinal rampage leaves in its wake a swath of interruptions and interferences among the body's natural systems and a traumatized landscape of dead and dying cells. Some of these interruptions and interferences are dangerous to your health, but all of them are necessary for your protection at this time.

If this was a television commercial, the helpful home/life/auto insurance agent would step forward about now and offer to help put right what has been ripped asunder. An adjuster is in order — but in this case, you need more than an estimate and a check. You need comforting, you need soothing, and you need practical suggestions on how to alleviate the seemingly endless string of side effects that chemotherapy can cause. Enter your oncologist and your chemo nurses. They have seen it all, heard it all, and come up with a seemingly endless string of possibilities that can help make your life easier as you undergo chemotherapy.

...s chapter, you find helpful hints for coping with the more serious side
...cts of chemotherapy, including nausea, fatigue, pain, depression, fertility
...blems, and hair loss.

Considering What's to Come

Chemotherapy has a way of undermining anything you may be vain about,
including your energy, your hearty appetite, your stamina, your smooth skin,
your hair, your quick wit, and even your ability to distinguish one cola drink
from another in a blind tasting. We are not here to debate the metaphysical
lessons that may be learned from such rigorous testing (and you may want to
avoid wandering into that hornet's nest as well). Instead, we're eager to
address ways that can help you compensate for these temporary losses.

Over time, almost everything you lose during chemotherapy comes back,
sometimes better than ever and sometimes good enough, all things
considered.

We explain in Chapters 4 and 8 why chemotherapy is an important weapon in
the battle against cancer, how it works, and how it affects your immune system.
When you're feeling overwhelmed by all the possible negative effects of this
course of treatment, take a look back at those chapters for reminders of the
very important positive outcomes that chemotherapy can bring.

If you've read Chapter 9, you know that many people develop side effects
from chemotherapy that are related to a drop in white blood cell counts, red
blood cell counts, and platelets. These side effects can lead directly to serious
infections and bleeding. (If you haven't read Chapter 9, we encourage you to
do so, because we offer advice for avoiding infection, trauma, and disease
while undergoing chemotherapy.)

Infections and bleeding aren't the only potential side effects, or risks, of
chemotherapy. Some side effects are more serious than others, but we fully
understand that you will take quite seriously any side effect that you experience. In other words, when we talk about "serious" side effects in this chapter and "less serious" side effects in Chapter 11, we understand that any side
effect you experience will be of concern. That's as it should be.

Specific side effects and their level of severity vary widely from person to
person and depend on factors such as the following:

- Your type of chemotherapy
- Your dose of chemotherapy
- Your body's reaction to chemotherapy
- Your general health

Each factor plays a part when it comes to determining which side effects you may experience.

Reading a firsthand report

While your coauthor Patricia was undergoing chemotherapy in 1995, she kept a journal documenting her experiences. Following is an excerpt concerning side effects.

Before you read this, she wants you to consider the context. Two weeks earlier, she attended a party at the Ritz-Carlton that lasted until midnight. She said she danced and laughed all night long "for the sheer joy of being among friends at a festive celebration." A month after she wrote this journal entry, she recorded that she felt much better and had started attending a support group at the St. Louis branch of The Wellness Community, a national cancer support organization that provides free services for people going through cancer treatments and their families. (See Chapter 17 for more information on support groups.)

Here is the journal entry:

> *My eyes are dry. My nose is dry. My lips are dry. My face is dry. All the rest of me is dry. Nothing tastes quite right. I'm tired. The muscles in my left upper arm hurt and I can't unhook my bra in the back. My vision is cloudy. My hair is all gone. My eyelashes are going. My eyebrows are half gone. My bones ache. This is all wearing me down, one side effect after another. I never want to go through this again.*

Months later, a friend told Patricia that she had read that cancer treatments "ravage" people. Our coauthor initially rejected that idea. "At first, I put up a brave front and insisted that I was only inconvenienced," she said. "At some point though, I admitted I was, indeed, ravaged."

Predicting your experience

Will you feel ravaged as a result of side effects from chemotherapy? We wish we could answer that question definitively and predict exactly which side effects you'll experience and to what extent, but we can't.

We hope that as you read this chapter, you can read it for information but not take every word personally. By that, we mean that sometimes, just knowing the full laundry list of possible side effects can cause a level of dismay that ranks right up there with some of the physical side effects. If you've ever been immunized for yellow fever or cholera before making a trip to a Third

World country, you know that right after you get the injection, you get a two- or three-page list of side effects that you may or may not suffer. Frankly, in that situation, it's best to skim over the list, tuck it into your pocket, and forget about it rather than dwell on what may or may not happen.

We won't suggest that you go that far in this case — we believe you're wise to want to be prepared for possible side effects when you begin chemotherapy. Still, you may want to carefully study what we have to say about any side effect listed here only if and when you experience it.

Keeping an Eye on Kidney and Bladder Function

You already know that chemotherapy drugs are strong medicine, so it may not come as a surprise to learn that these drugs sometimes irritate the bladder or even damage the bladder and kidneys. Sometimes the damage is temporary; sometimes it is permanent. If you are on one of the drugs known for causing side effects in the kidney and bladder, your doctor may ask you from time to time to collect a urine sample over 24 hours.

Some chemotherapy drugs can cause your urine to appear a different color than usual and to exude a medicinal odor for a day or two. Most likely, your doctor will alert you if you are taking one of these drugs.

Symptoms that may indicate a problem with the kidneys or bladder include

- ✔ Pain or burning during urination
- ✔ Frequent urination
- ✔ Inability to urinate
- ✔ Urgent need to urinate
- ✔ Reddish or bloody urine
- ✔ Fever
- ✔ Chills that give you the shakes

If any of these symptoms occur, be sure to call your doctor. And no matter what kind of chemotherapy you are undergoing, remember to drink plenty of fluids. You have many choices, including

- ✔ Water
- ✔ Juice
- ✔ Soft drinks

> ✔ Broth
>
> ✔ Ice cream
>
> ✔ Soup
>
> ✔ Popsicles
>
> ✔ Gelatin

Good fluid intake moves the anticancer drugs through your system and also ensures good urine flow.

Combating Nausea

A few decades ago, nausea and vomiting were real problems for people undergoing chemotherapy. Today, much better anti-nausea drugs — and a much wider variety of them — are available.

If you feel queasy after chemotherapy and you think the anti-nausea medication that you're taking is not doing its job, speak up. Talk with your doctor or chemo nurse about trying a different drug. If that one doesn't work for you either, report in again and switch to a different medication. It may take some experimenting, or you may get it right the first time, but we know for certain that drugs are available that can control any nausea and vomiting.

If you haven't hit on the best anti-nausea drug for you just yet — or even if you have — the following sections contain some practical suggestions that can help you avoid nausea.

Eating smart

Obviously, if you're experiencing nausea you want to pay close attention to what — and how — you eat. The following suggestions can help:

- ✔ **Eat before you get up in the morning.** Try a couple crackers or some dry cereal so you have something in your stomach before you start your day. You can put the crackers on a bedside table each night before you go to bed.

- ✔ **Avoid spicy foods.** Tacos, curries, and pepper steak come to mind. Other no-no's include greasy foods and any foods with strong odors that may unsettle your stomach. One way to avoid cooking odors, of course, is to eat only cold foods.

- ✔ **Take small bites.** Also, chew your food thoroughly.

✔ **Eat several small meals.** Spreading your meals throughout the day ensures that you never have an empty stomach.

✔ **Take in some protein.** Get the biggest nutritional bang for your buck by eating foods such as eggs, tuna, or peanut butter. However, if these foods seem to upset your stomach, stick to high-carbohydrate foods such as rice, pasta, or potatoes.

✔ **Stay away from sweets.** The rich desserts, doughnuts, and Danish rolls will have to wait.

Drinking smart

Here's the catch: Dehydration and over-hydration both induce nausea, so you need to try to balance the amount of fluid that's in your stomach at any given time. Here are some tips:

✔ **Sip small amounts.** It may take conscious effort at first, but you need to learn not to swallow too much at a time.

✔ **Drink from a straw.** This is one way to insure that you don't drink too much at a time.

✔ **Drink only liquids at room temperature.** Anything too hot or too cold may upset your stomach.

✔ **Drink before and after meals instead of while you eat.** Sending down food or liquid one at a time works better than combining the two.

✔ **Stick to unsweetened fruit juices.** Clear juices, such as apple, are best if you like juice better than water.

✔ **Defizz carbonated drinks.** If you've got a craving for soda, try a few sips of a clear carbonated beverage — such as ginger ale — that has been allowed to go flat.

✔ **Settle in with a cup of herbal tea.** Remember to drink it warm, not hot. Peppermint tea is known for soothing the stomach.

✔ **Avoid caffeinated drinks.** Caffeine is a powerful drug in and of itself, and if you are feeling woozy, the caffeine may make you feel worse.

Comforting yourself

If, despite your best efforts, you still have to cope with occasional nausea, you can find ways to comfort yourself when you're not feeling well. Here are some strategies:

- ✔ **Remove tight clothing.** This is the time to wrap yourself in an old, cozy bathrobe or climb into your favorite stretched-out sweats.

- ✔ **Take deep, slow breaths.** Concentrate on your breathing to keep it even, and try to relax any tight muscles, especially in your stomach.

- ✔ **Strap on a wristband.** People worried about seasickness on cruises wear wristbands that touch acupressure points. You can find these wristbands at your local pharmacy.

- ✔ **Suck on ice chips.** Or, if you prefer to suck on hard candy, try peppermint or lemon drops.

- ✔ **Put a cold cloth over your eyes.** Try lying down for 30 minutes (unless you've just eaten).

- ✔ **Get plenty of rest.** If you can relax enough to have a nap, you likely will feel better when you wake up.

Facing Fatigue

Advising someone undergoing chemotherapy to get a lot of rest really isn't necessary. The level of fatigue you're likely to face during treatments will send you off to bed uncharacteristically early and perhaps even result in a new fascination with naps.

This is a fatigue like no other. In fact, the word *fatigue* doesn't do justice to this experience. You've certainly been tired in your life, and you've probably experienced what you thought was fatigue. When that's happened, you've gone to bed early, gotten some rest, and bounced right back. During chemotherapy, what you most likely will experience — as reported by 70 percent of people on anticancer drugs — is exhaustion from the inside out. This exhaustion is ever present, though it occasionally varies in degree. No matter how much sleep you get, it may never be enough.

Some researchers blame fatigue on the fluctuating red blood cell count that occurs during chemotherapy. After all, red blood cells take oxygen from the lungs and move it throughout the body, providing energy. Anticancer drugs cause your body to produce fewer red blood cells, so it makes sense that you would have less energy. But stress may play a part as well — both the emotional stress of dealing with cancer and the physical stress of undergoing treatment while still attempting to maintain a semblance of normal life.

So you're tired — even tired beyond tired. What can you do?

Checking for anemia

First things first. Tell your doctor that you're tired and that the fatigue is having an impact on everything you try to do. With a simple blood test, your doctor can determine if you have anemia, which is a decreased red blood cell count. If you do, your doctor can advise if it needs to be treated with a colony stimulating factor (see Chapter 9) or a blood transfusion.

Conserving energy

You also want to safeguard whatever energy you do have and make the most of it. To conserve your energy, first we recommend that you learn to say "no." This word is especially important when you're just starting to undergo chemotherapy and learning what you can and can't do and how to find the balance in between.

Let's practice. Face yourself in the mirror and repeat saying "no" until it loses all power to make you feel guilty, ashamed, or somehow less than you are. "No" is a perfectly legitimate word and an exceptionally powerful tool if you truly want to conserve your energy.

When you are tired, use this word whenever you or anyone else asks you to do anything that can be put off until later, anything that really doesn't have to be done ever, anything that someone else could easily do for you, or anything that you sense will send you over the edge into total exhaustion. Saying "no" to someone else often is a way of saying "yes" to yourself.

Here are some additional tips to safeguard the energy you do have:

✔ **Pace yourself.** If you are working full-time or even part-time while undergoing chemotherapy, you know you need to give much of your energy to your employer. Still, save some back so you will be able to enjoy family activities and time spent with friends. If you know you will be busy Thursday night, plan to take it easy on Wednesday evening. If Sunday is a big day for you, lie low on Saturday. Take into account on a day-to-day basis how much energy you have and divide it up accordingly. That two-letter word comes in handy here.

✔ **Change your pace.** Some days, your energy may last well into evening before serious fatigue sets in. Some days, you'll be ready to call it quits by midafternoon. And some days, morning will come and you will have nothing to offer the day in terms of energy. Change your pace accordingly. A famous 12-step program advises taking it one day at a time. When you're being treated for cancer, feel free to take it a half day at a time. If that's the best you can do, that's more than sufficient.

✔ **Plan your day.** Each morning, write down or make a mental lis you hope to accomplish in the course of the day. You should kno away if you are expecting too much of yourself. If so, reassign som tasks to another day or — even better — to another person.

✔ **Include naps or breaks in your plan.** No daily plan is complete withou one or more opportunities for short naps or breaks. Now, you may not think of yourself as a person who takes naps. However, during chemotherapy, you may inadvertently turn into one of those people. If you stretch out on a couch or lean back in an easy chair to rest your eyes for a minute, you may easily slip into a full-fledged nap that lasts 20 to 30 minutes. Good for you!

✔ **Get a little exercise.** Research has shown that even a short walk can help decrease fatigue. That may sound crazy, and you may think that exercise will make you even more tired. You may be right. On the other hand, just a little exercise each day may bring you some renewed energy.

✔ **Fuel the body.** Even when your health is at its peak, your body requires fuel to function efficiently. Be sure you are eating a nutritious diet. (For more information, see Chapter 15.) Protein and carbohydrates, particularly, provide essential fuels.

✔ **Consider complementary therapies.** Some people find that fatigue decreases if they practice guided meditation or guided imagery or spend some time in prayer. (See Chapters 14 and 16 for more on these therapies.)

It's all just a game

In 2004, a 9-year-old former leukemia patient was the source of inspiration for a video game that helps people undergoing cancer treatments take their minds off the side effects of chemotherapy. Ben Duskin of San Francisco told Associated Press writer Paul Elias that when the Make-A-Wish Foundation approached him, he wanted to do "something special, something more than going on a Disney cruise and stuff like that."

An engineer at LucasArts who creates video games volunteered to help Ben, and together, they developed "Ben's Game." According to Elias, the game's central character "zooms around the screen on a skateboard, zapping mutated cells and collecting seven shields to protect against common side effects of chemotherapy, which include nausea, hair loss and fevers." The game was officially unveiled at the University of California's San Francisco Pediatric Treatment Center.

Fighting Pain

Some anticancer drugs affect the nerves. The result may be muscles that are weak or sore. Your feet or legs may hurt when you walk. Individual body parts may tremble or shake. Some drugs cause painful mouth sores. And sometimes chemotherapy can lead to headaches or stomach pain.

Just as your doctor has a wide range of anti-nausea drugs that can help you, she also can help alleviate pain. Be sure to communicate clearly to your doctor what you're experiencing, and don't hesitate to ask for help with pain relief.

Some symptoms of pain are more serious than others, but all are worthy of reporting to your doctor. This information will help your doctor help you:

- ✔ Where is the pain?
- ✔ What kind of pain is it?
- ✔ How strong is the pain?
- ✔ How long does the pain last?

If you do go on medication for pain, keep in touch with your doctor so she knows how it's working and whether you are getting the help you need.

People who are reluctant to take pain medication are sometimes inclined to skip a dose here and there or stop the medication altogether when the pain eases up. Usually, that's a mistake. Pain medication works best on a cumulative basis. Generally, the drug needs to build up in your system to a level where it can make a significant difference in your pain. If you skip every other dose or decide to stop taking your pills after two days, you'll quickly be back to square one, calling the doctor again to complain about your pain.

Keep in mind that the "recommended dose" for pain medication is recommended for a reason. Have a little faith, and take the drugs as instructed.

Nailing neuropathy

Neuropathy is another word for nerve damage. Early symptoms include tingling, numbness, or a burning sensation in the fingers and toes. Over time, neuropathy may cause you to lose your sense of touch, and you may have difficulty performing fine motor tasks such as buttoning a shirt or picking up a coffee cup. Sometimes, constipation results from neuropathy.

If you experience any of these symptoms, talk with your doctor. If the neuropathy continues to progress or spread, the doctor may recommend medication or physical therapy. In some cases, your doctor may lower your dose of your current chemotherapy or switch you to a different anticancer drug altogether. If you develop pain as a result of neuropathy, your doctor may prescribe an analgesic or other medication. The most important thing you can do is take the pain medication prescribed by your doctor — on time and on a regular basis.

Watching out for mouth sores

Sores that develop in the mouth or throat during chemotherapy can be very painful. Sometimes, the sores become infected because our warm, moist mouths are havens for many kinds of bacteria. These infections are harder to fight because chemotherapy interferes with the optimal function of the immune system (see Chapter 9).

Also, chemotherapy can cause the protective cells that line the tissues of the mouth and throat to become *devitalized,* or scraped raw, much as you remove a thin layer of skin when you scrape a knee or elbow against a hard surface. Sometimes, the sores even bleed because the tissue is dry and irritated. Almost always, mouth and throat sores lead to a decrease in appetite because, well, it hurts to eat. That said, this is no time to give up eating. Good nutrition is vital while undergoing chemotherapy.

In this situation, the old adage "An ounce of prevention is worth a pound of cure" rules the day. Even before you begin chemotherapy, you want to practice the highest level of oral hygiene.

Preventing mouth and throat sores

When you first learn that you will undergo chemotherapy, call your dentist and schedule an appointment to take place before your anticancer treatments begin. Have your teeth cleaned, and ask the dentist to attend to any cavities or other problems. Sometimes, people develop more cavities than usual while on chemotherapy, so ask if you need to consider any fluoride-rich gels or pastes to help protect yourself. Ask, too, for a refresher course in the best way to brush and floss your teeth. (Have you ever met a dental hygienist who would be less than thrilled with such a request?) Most of us get lazy about oral hygiene from time to time, but this is not the time.

Here are some tips on how to care for your mouth and throat during chemotherapy:

- ✔ Rinse your mouth with warm saltwater after each meal and before bedtime.
- ✔ Brush your teeth and gums after every meal.
- ✔ Use a brush with soft bristles.
- ✔ Brush thoroughly, but don't use a heavy hand.
- ✔ Use a special toothpaste if your gums are particularly sensitive.
- ✔ Rinse your toothbrush after each use and store it where it can dry.
- ✔ Use a mouthwash that does not contain alcohol.

Treating mouth and throat sores

Even if you practice perfect oral hygiene, sores may develop in your mouth and throat. Some medications are available that you apply directly to mouth sores. Other medications, in pill form, may also help. Be sure to ask your doctor about these options.

When mouth and throat sores develop, eating can become a challenge. Here are some tips to make eating less painful:

- ✔ Eat foods that are cold or at room temperature; avoid hot or even warm foods.
- ✔ Eat soft foods that soothe the throat — think ice cream, applesauce, mashed potatoes (hold the garlic), oatmeal, scrambled eggs, yogurt, cottage cheese, pudding, or gelatin.
- ✔ Stay away from acidic fruits and juices, such as citrus (orange, lemon, grapefruit) and tomato.
- ✔ Avoid all spicy or salty foods.
- ✔ Save rough or coarse foods (raw vegetables, popcorn, toast) until after your mouth heals.

Dealing with dry mouth

Even if you escape developing mouth sores, anticancer drugs may cause your mouth to dry out, which can be very uncomfortable. Your doctor may recommend an artificial saliva product to help moisten your mouth. Here are some other tips:

- ✔ Drink plenty of liquids.
- ✔ Suck on ice chips, Popsicles, lemon drops, or other hard candy to stimulate saliva production.

- ✔ Avoid dry foods or moisten them with butter, sauce, or broth.
- ✔ Eat soft foods.
- ✔ Carry a lip balm and moisten your lips often.

Demystifying Depression

Not all pain is physical. Being diagnosed with cancer also can cause emotional pain and even extreme anxiety and depression. You may worry how you got cancer and how you will cope with the diagnosis and treatment. You most assuredly will worry — or at least wonder with great intensity — whether your treatments will be successful and you will survive.

Facing your fear

The moment when you fully realize that you may not live forever, as you (and the rest of us) had planned — when you realize that indeed cancer may carry you off long before you are prepared to go — is a difficult moment. Faced with that moment, many people find themselves mentally zipping through several of the stages of grief documented by author Elizabeth Kubler-Ross. Those stages are

- ✔ Denial
- ✔ Anger
- ✔ Bargaining
- ✔ Despair
- ✔ Acceptance

What causes this fear of our mortality to abate? It's the surprising — and somewhat embarrassing — revelation that people with cancer are not the only people left in the dark on this very personal and important matter. No one gets a guarantee. Really, all you can do from this moment on is vow to live now and to live better. We share some thoughts on this important topic in Chapters 20 and 24.

Identifying other causes of depression

The changes that chemotherapy causes to your body — not to mention to your life — also can cause depression. Some of these feelings occur when the anticancer drugs interfere with some functions of your central nervous system or brain. Some of them occur, frankly, because going through cancer treatments can be depressing. Some level of depression is normal (although it's still disturbing). Deeper levels of depression may signal a need for professional help.

Getting the help you need

If you have a case of the blues, you can first try to elevate your own mood. Here are some suggestions:

- ✔ See a funny movie.
- ✔ Read a funny book.
- ✔ Listen to music you love.
- ✔ Make cookies for an elderly neighbor.
- ✔ Buy a CD that teaches beginning Italian.
- ✔ Go for a short walk.
- ✔ Work a crossword puzzle.
- ✔ Snuggle with your cat or dog.

Don't laugh at that last one: Research has shown that stroking a beloved pet elevates mood. But if you and your pet can't beat the blues together, talk to a family member or close friend. Speak with your doctor. Investigate support groups or one-on-one peer counseling available to you. (For information about support groups, see Chapter 17.)

If you think your blues have reached a point where you would welcome more support than pets, family, friends, or a support group can provide, speak with your doctor. Don't wait for someone else to make the first move. No one knows better than you how you feel and how you are coping emotionally with cancer treatments. Help is readily available; if you need it, do yourself a favor and speak up. Some symptoms of depression that indicate a call for help include

- ✔ Withdrawal from other people
- ✔ Decreased appetite
- ✔ Heightened sense of anger
- ✔ Feelings of hopelessness
- ✔ Uneven sleep patterns
- ✔ Lack of personal hygiene
- ✔ Loss of any pleasure in pleasurable activities

Your doctor can recommend trained counseling professionals who can help you cope with your feelings. Among the options are

- Psychiatrists
- Psychologists
- Social workers
- Clergy
- Counselors trained especially to work with people going through cancer treatments

If necessary, your doctor (or a psychiatrist) may recommend medications to help lift depression. If you do decide to take medication, talk with your medical oncologist first to make sure that the drug will not interfere with chemotherapy treatments.

Confronting Infertility

Your central nervous system and immune system are not the only systems affected by chemotherapy. Anticancer drugs also alter the reproductive system. Put in plainer terms, some chemotherapy drugs cause infertility. Depending on the drug and your age, the infertility may be temporary or it may be permanent, and there is no way to know for sure at the outset.

In men, chemotherapy may lower the number of sperm cells or restrict the sperm from moving freely. Other possible side effects are erectile dysfunction and chromosomal damage, which could cause birth defects. In women, anticancer drugs may damage the ovaries. Some women experience a *pseudo menopause,* complete with irregular (or completely stopped) menstrual periods, hot flashes, and vaginal dryness. Again, these changes may be temporary, or they may be permanent. (Read more about long-term effects of cancer treatments in Chapter 19.)

For some people, especially younger people, this information about the potentially permanent loss of fertility immediately causes a deep sense of loss. Others react later, after treatments are complete. Still others concentrate on beating cancer and accept this side effect as a necessary loss. There is no one correct response.

Being proactive

We urge you not to guess about your reaction or that of your spouse or partner. Make an appointment with your oncologist so the three of you may talk about this serious topic before your first chemotherapy treatment. Talk about your feelings and discuss your options. Some men choose to open an account, as it were, at a sperm bank. Some women choose to store unfertilized eggs, which are frozen until needed. The fertilization rate of frozen eggs later is not high, but research continues. Research also is underway regarding the viability of freezing ovarian tissue and later returning it to the woman in the hope that she may bear a child, but the procedure is not available in most medical centers, as it is still the subject of active investigation.

Planning to wait

If you had hoped to have a baby in the near future — whether you are a woman or a man — you need to put that hope on hold. Harsh chemotherapy drugs can affect the growth and development of a fetus, so you need to avoid pregnancy until your treatments are over. If you are a woman taking anticancer drugs, it's easy to understand the risk. If you are a man undergoing chemotherapy, the drugs can show up in sperm, so the risk to the fetus is also very real.

No matter which partner is undergoing chemotherapy, use reliable contraception at all times. If you are a woman taking birth control pills, ask your doctor whether the pills will interfere with anticancer drugs or if you should switch to another form of birth control. Even after chemotherapy is over, it's best to wait a bit before trying to conceive, just to be certain all the drugs are out of your system.

If you are pregnant when you are diagnosed with cancer, your options depend on several factors, including

- The type of cancer
- The stage of the cancer
- The treatments recommended
- The stage of the pregnancy
- Your desire to bear a child at this time

Sometimes, if you are in the later stages of pregnancy, treatment can be delayed or offered at a lower dose. Speak with your doctor. If ever there was a case where one size does not fit all, this is it.

Losing Your Hair

When you compare losing your hair to experiencing nausea, fatigue, pain, depression, and fertility problems, it doesn't sound so bad, does it? Still, hair loss — even though it is strictly temporary — ranks high on the list of side

Expecting changes in your love life

Cancer changes everything, and your sex life is no exception. Going through cancer treatments takes a toll physically and emotionally, so you should expect one of two things to happen regarding intimacy: It will get better, or it will get worse. It may get better because going through cancer together can increase a sense of teamwork in a couple. You both may display affection more freely and quite literally cling to one another. This heightened sense of partnership may lead to more sexual expression as well. On the other hand, the partner going through treatments may fret about changes in appearance or simply feel wiped out much of the time. These circumstances may lead to less interest in sex.

We are happy to report that there likely will be no lack of interest in cuddling. The gentle touch; the kind and encouraging words; and the accompanying sense of comfort, acceptance, and peace are almost always welcome.

effects that cause emotional distress among both men and women. More accurately, the *process* of losing of your hair is particularly upsetting. After it's gone, most people adapt, but from the moment it first starts falling out until you sweep up the last of it, you may have a hard time emotionally.

In Chapter 8, we explain that you may find your first chemotherapy treatment anticlimactic when compared to the level of anxiety that precedes it. But there is something about your hair falling out that makes the whole experience of cancer treatments and what you will face in the coming months more real than ever.

Some types of chemotherapy cause only thinning of the hair, and some cause total hair loss. Either way, your hair will grow back after treatments end.

Hair loss (also known as *alopecia*) occurs sometime after the first or second chemotherapy treatment. If you are under the impression that only the hair on your head will be affected, think again. You may lose your eyelashes, eyebrows, any facial hair, the hair on your legs and arms, and hair in your pubic area. (Or, in a cruel twist of fate, only the hair on your legs may decide to stick around so that — if you're a woman — you may still feel obligated to shave your legs.)

Caring for your hair before it goes

While you still have hair, you want to treat it differently than before you started chemotherapy. Here are some tips that will help keep your hair — and your scalp — healthy:

- ✔ Invest in a mild shampoo.
- ✔ Brush your hair with soft strokes using a soft hairbrush.
- ✔ Hold off on dying, perming, or relaxing your hair.
- ✔ Put away the brush rollers.
- ✔ Use only the low setting on your hair dryer.

These precautions simply help you protect yourself from infections. Like the rest of your skin, your scalp will be more sensitive during chemotherapy.

Planning ahead for hair loss

Because hair loss is such an emotional experience (for men as well as women), spend some time getting used to the idea of yourself without hair. Wigs, hats, and scarves all are available (see Figure 10-1), so think about what head covering(s) you will use — if any — and what else you can do to maintain a positive body image after your hair is gone. For obvious reasons, this is easier to do before you lose your hair.

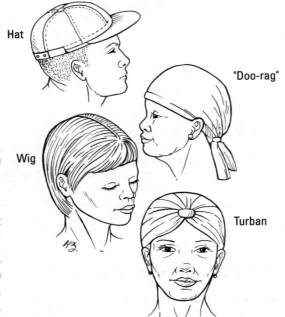

Figure 10-1: Consider whether you want to use hats, scarves, wigs, or turbans if you lose your hair.

Choosing a wig

If you are a woman, think about whether you will want a wig. If you want a wig and you think you will prefer to recognize yourself in the mirror, visit a wig shop before your hair falls out so you can match your current style and color. You may think that visiting the wig shop will be a grim expedition. It doesn't have to be. We recommend that you take a friend who makes you laugh, and then go out for lunch afterward. You may even decide to try a wig that is a totally new style and color of hair for you. If price is not an issue, get two!

Most insurance companies pay for one wig — which they call a *prosthesis* — for people undergoing chemotherapy. If your insurance company will not pay for a wig or you don't have insurance, contact your local branch of the American Cancer Society. Women who have recovered from cancer often donate their wigs and other head coverings, and these are available for free. Also, some medical centers have a wig "exchange" where you can find an attractive covering for your head.

Wigs can be made from human hair (which is very expensive) or from synthetic hair (which is much more reasonably priced).

Sometimes, wigs cause a rash on the scalp, especially in summer when your scalp perspires under the wig. The best way to treat this rash is to expose your bald head to the open air as often as possible. Rub on a mild, over-the-counter cortisone cream if needed. When you want to wear the wig, place a piece of clean cotton fabric between your scalp and your wig — an old, well-washed bandanna, folded to fit, is perfect. It won't show, and the cotton will absorb the moisture that caused the rash.

Caring for a wig

All wigs, even expensive ones, require some care. They look best if they're kept on a Styrofoam wig head when not in use. (Our coauthor Patricia propped hers up on a potato chip container and referred to her wig as "Mrs. Pringle's hair.")

Wigs tend to look more natural when they're fluffed up to more closely resemble real hair. If you don't have magic fingers and your wig resists your fluffing efforts, speak with your hairdresser. He may be willing to take ten minutes to tend to your wig once a week or for special occasions, depending on how much this matters to you.

Depending on how many months you have to wear the wig, you likely will want to wash it a time or two. This isn't hard, but it's not always easy to get the wig back to looking like it should. You use warm water and a mild detergent soap, swish the wig around for a bit, rinse it several times, dry it with a towel, and put it back on your wig stand or potato chip container. For more detailed instructions and tips on how to fluff it back up, talk with the sales clerk at the wig shop.

If these remedies do not help, speak with your doctor because there are other options, depending upon the appearance of the rash.

Choosing an alternative head covering

A wig is not your only option:

- ✔ Some women prefer to wear a scarf or turban instead of a wig after they lose their hair.

- ✔ Most men — and a few women — go about with bald pate gleaming. Will people stare? Some may; if they do, just flash a confident smile and go on your way. Going "topless," as it were, is fine for indoors.

  If your bare head gets cold at night, consider buying or making a stretchy, cotton knit cap that will keep your head warm and your dreams in place.

- ✔ Some people invest in a signature hat to wear outdoors to protect their bald scalps from sunburn, which is important all the time but especially so during cancer treatments.

All these decisions are personal, so do whatever feels right for you. There are no rules except those you make, and you can always change the rules to suit yourself.

Cutting your hair

You may want to make an appointment to have your hair cut short. This proactive approach provides you with an emotional way station between having a full head of hair and none at all. If all your hair comes out, it's easier to manage losing short hair than long — for a while, anyway. And if only a little of your hair ends up falling out, the hair that is left will look thicker and fuller if it's short.

Hair falls out in single strands and in clumps. Once it starts coming out, hair will lie on your pillow, litter your collar, and coat the walls of your shower. Frankly, it's a mess — such a mess that you may find yourself dialing your hair stylist and asking for an appointment to have your head shaved.

If you suspect that you may become weepy while having your head shaved, ask if you can schedule the appointment after hours or if there is a private room where you can get the job done and then don your wig or head covering before leaving the salon. Keep in mind that you are not the first person to make this type of call, and you will not be the last. Most stylists are happy to do what they can to help you through this difficult appointment.

Replacing eyebrows and lashes

Whether to replace your eyebrows and lashes is a personal decision: Some women choose not to bother, and some feel comforted when they look in the mirror and see the eyebrows and lashes they expect to see.

If you are a woman accustomed to running an eyebrow pencil over your brows to thicken or darken them, you may do fine when it comes time to draw them on from scratch. If you've never owned an eyebrow pencil, you may want to buy one before treatment begins and pay attention to that bony arch above each eye. That's where the brow goes. Usually, a natural brow starts out fairly thick near the bridge of the nose, thickens slightly right above the iris and then tapers off on the other side. You can actually buy a set of eyebrow stencils and play around, seeing what shape suits you. Some people opt for permanent cosmetics, or tattooed eyebrows. If that interests you, make an appointment before your eyelashes fall out so the aesthetician can match the color and shape of your natural brows.

As for eyelashes, you could invest in a pair of false eyelashes or glue on false lashes one at a time, though that strikes us as a lot of trouble. You could also put a little eyeliner on the edge of each upper and lower lid. Another option is tattooed eyeliner, which you would have forever.

"Look Good, Feel Better" (www.lookgoodfeelbetter.org) is a national public service program founded in 1989 to help women with their makeup and wigs while going through chemotherapy. Many hospitals present workshops conducted by representatives of this program.

If your medical center does not have such a program and you want help drawing on eyebrows or putting on makeup, stride boldly into a nearby department store and ask one of the makeup consultants at the cosmetics counter to help you. This service is free. Also, we offer additional tips about skin care and makeup in Chapter 11.

Growing new hair

Here's the good news: Four to six weeks after your last chemotherapy treatment, your hair follicles will recover and begin to produce hair. Typically, hair grows about a quarter inch per month. When your hair first comes back in, you may think it's someone else's hair. If you had curly hair, it may come in straight. If you had straight hair, you may end up with a head full of curls. The texture may be different, and your new hair may show up in a shade of rodent gray that really doesn't suit you at all.

Be patient. After growing for three or four months, your hair may revert to the texture and color you expected. If it doesn't, this is no time to break out a bottle of sparkling burgundy hair color bought at the grocery. This is new hair on your head — delicate, fragile, baby-soft hair. Soon the day will come — maybe six months from that first growth — when you can color, perm, or even straighten your hair so you will truly feel like yourself again. Or, you may decide you prefer your new look.

Meanwhile, treat your new hair gently. And think about this: Eventually, the day will come when your hair will be long and scraggly, and you will make an appointment to have it cut. Imagine that!

Chapter 11

Coping with Less Serious Side Effects of Chemotherapy

· ·

In This Chapter
▶ Experiencing intestinal upsets
▶ Coping with blurred vision
▶ Fighting fuzzy thinking
▶ Losing your appetite
▶ Making the most of moisturizing

· ·

*W*ouldn't you think that low blood counts, nausea, fatigue, pain, depression, fertility problems, and hair loss would be plenty of side effects for any one anticancer drug to cause?

Yes, you would — but you would be wrong.

Ever vigilant, moving along every main road and into every back alley of the body, chemotherapy drugs have such an impact on every system that we have to use three chapters just to fit in all the potential side effects. In Chapter 9, we discuss low blood counts and how to avoid infection, trauma, and disease while taking anticancer drugs. In Chapter 10, we address the additional serious side effects caused by chemotherapy's interference with all the body's operating systems. Here, we take up the less serious side effects.

We understand that any side effect you experience will be of intense concern, and that's as it should be. We also know that one person interprets a particular side effect as devastating while another person who experiences the same side effect considers it merely annoying. Still, none of the side effects we discuss in this chapter are life threatening. Like all risks and side effects from chemotherapy, most of those included here are temporary, and your doctor can help you find solutions to them. Also, when pondering all the risks and side effects of chemotherapy, you want to remember that the positive effects of chemotherapy include tumor shrinkage, disease-free survival, and overall survival of cancer. That likely will make the price you pay seem worth the trouble.

In this chapter, you find helpful hints for coping with the less serious side effects of chemotherapy, including diarrhea, constipation, fluid retention, vision problems, "chemo brain," loss of appetite, and a variety of skin problems.

When it comes to side effects of chemotherapy, here is our wish for you: May they all be "less serious" in nature — and if they are not, may it help to think of them in that way.

Considering What's to Come

As we say in Chapter 10, we cannot predict which side effects from chemotherapy you will experience. You may get a good number of them, or you may get none — most likely, your experience will be somewhere in between. Specific side effects and their level of severity vary widely from person to person. Factors to consider include

- Your type of chemotherapy
- Your dose of chemotherapy
- Your body's reaction to chemotherapy
- Your general health
- Miscellaneous, unpredictable reactions

All these factors play a part when it comes to determining which side effects you may experience. Here then, are some of the possibilities.

Battling Intestinal Disarray

This isn't fair or particularly logical, but some chemotherapy drugs can cause diarrhea and others can cause constipation. (Sometimes, pain medication can cause intestinal disarray, but since you're taking these drugs only because you're undergoing chemotherapy, it's all part of the same package.) Let's look at these conditions one at a time.

Dealing with diarrhea

Maybe it's too much garlic in the pasta sauce, or maybe you're a tad lactose intolerant. Or maybe the watery or loose stools result when your anticancer drugs encounter the cells lining your intestine.

Actually, you don't have to know why you get diarrhea. You do need to pay attention to how long the diarrhea lasts, because over time, it can lead to dehydration and other serious complications. If it goes on for more than 24 hours, or if you have pain and cramping, you want to call your doctor.

Resist taking any over-the-counter medication before you make the call, as your doctor may have something stronger in mind. Also, if the diarrhea shows no signs of stopping, if you are more than 65 years old, or if you normally take medications to lower your blood pressure, the doctor may recommend intravenous fluids to replace the water and nutrients you have lost. That's a simple treatment, usually done as an outpatient procedure.

Some specific chemotherapy drugs cause diarrhea or give you a predisposition to an infection with a diarrhea-causing organism. If you are to be treated with such a drug, your doctor will tell you so before treatments begin and prescribe drugs for you to take as soon as the diarrhea starts.

If the cause of diarrhea is something other than your anticancer drug, you probably already have some ideas on how to control it and help care for yourself at the same time. Here are some tips:

- **Drink, drink, drink.** Mild, clear liquids are best — think water, broth, ginger ale, or a sports drink — served at room temperature. If you're drinking ginger ale or a citrus-flavored soft drink, pour it in a glass and wait until the drink goes flat. Stay away from fruit juices for now.

- **Eat small meals throughout the day.** Low-fiber foods are best, including white rice, noodles, mashed or baked potatoes, fish, and skinless chicken or turkey. Stay away from high-fiber foods such as whole grain breads, cereal, beans, nuts, seeds, popcorn, raw vegetables, and any kind of fresh or dried fruit. Lay off milk products for now as well.

- **Take in some potassium.** You lose potassium when you have diarrhea, so help to replace it by eating bananas, oranges, and potatoes. Peach and apricot nectars both are good sources of potassium, too, so if you find them appealing, drink up.

Dealing with constipation

Sometimes, constipation is a result of chemotherapy drugs or pain medication. You also probably are less active than you were before your diagnosis, and you may not be eating enough fiber.

Regardless of the cause, constipation is a problem that can be resolved. If it goes on for more than two days, you want to call your doctor. Resist taking any over-the-counter medication before you make the call, as your doctor may want to check your white blood cell count or platelet count before prescribing a laxative or stool softener.

More than likely, you experienced constipation at some point before you were diagnosed with cancer, so you probably already have some ideas on how to proceed and help care for yourself at the same time. Here are some tips:

- **Drink, drink, drink.** Fluids in your system help loosen the bowels. If you aren't troubled by mouth sores, warm or hot fluids work especially well.

- **Boost your fiber intake.** Check with your doctor first, because fiber may present a problem for certain kinds of cancer and some side effects. If you get the go-ahead, make sure your diet includes bran, whole-wheat bread, whole-grain cereal, raw and cooked vegetables, fresh and dried fruits, nuts, and popcorn.

- **Exercise each day.** We're not suggesting you head to the gym for a three-hour workout, but a short walk each day may put an end to the constipation and also give you a bit more energy.

Retaining Fluids

If you aren't plagued with diarrhea or constipation, you may notice swelling or puffiness in your face, hands, feet, or abdomen. This swelling occurs when the body retains fluids. Why are you retaining fluids? Well, the chemotherapy may be to blame. It could be hormonal changes caused by chemotherapy. Or maybe it's a symptom of your cancer.

Don't guess: Call your doctor, talk about the problem, and see what he suggests. You may need to cut back on table salt or avoid it altogether. Or a *diuretic* — a medication that helps your body get rid of excess fluid — may be in order.

Experiencing Vision Problems

Some anticancer drugs may cause vision problems. The good news is that most of these problems go away a few days after each treatment, or certainly after all your treatments have ended. Still, if you have vision problems while undergoing chemotherapy, you do need to report them to your doctor and monitor them. Here are some symptoms to watch for:

✔ Cloudy vision

✔ Blurred vision

✔ Sudden loss of vision

✔ Sensitivity to light

✔ Severe eye pain

If you experience any of these symptoms, you want to call your doctor. Chemotherapy drugs are capable of causing everything from dry eyes to an increased risk of cataracts, so it's best not to ignore any symptoms of vision problems. You may need an antibiotic to counteract conjunctivitis (also known as *pink eye*), or you may need eye drops to help keep your eyes better lubricated. Your doctor will know.

Fighting Fuzzy Thinking

Sometimes, it's not just your vision that gets fuzzy during treatments. In Chapter 10, we mention that chemotherapy has a way of undermining anything you may be vain about, including a sharp intellect or quick wit. People who have experienced this reduction in brainpower refer to it as *chemo brain*. Basically, some people report that anticancer drugs leave them feeling "fuzzy" and somewhat confused, as if they have jet lag — without the benefit of the European vacation! Others complain of short-term memory loss.

The joke here, which may or may not strike you as funny, is that maybe your doctor warned you ahead of time about short-term memory loss, but after chemotherapy, you may not recall the conversation!

For years, many doctors attributed these symptoms to anything and everything but chemotherapy. Not any longer. At a conference held in Orlando, Florida, in 2004, researchers from the University of California at Los Angeles presented imaging studies that showed "marked differences in the brains of breast-cancer patients who had undergone chemotherapy compared to patients who had undergone surgery alone." Cognitive problems related to "focus, fast thinking, organization skills and an inability to multitask" have also been reported in individuals with other cancers, including lymphoma and lung cancer.

Tim A. Ahles, Ph.D., program director of the center of psycho-oncology research at Dartmouth Medical School, has led much of the recent research on this subject. He reports that nearly two-thirds of women treated with chemotherapy for breast cancer develop some level of cognitive problems. Most of these women recover several months after treatment ends, but as many as 20 to 25 percent develop lasting problems. Researchers and doctors alike make the point that though *chemo brain* can be frustrating, it is manageable, even when it sticks around. Research, of course, continues.

Losing Interest in Food

Temporarily losing your reputation for being sharp as a tack is one thing. That can be frustrating and sometimes, especially at work, even slightly embarrassing. Losing your appetite can have more serious ramifications. The best thing you can do to help your body cope with the powerful chemotherapy drugs coursing through you is eat a balanced diet that offers plenty of good nutrition. You need calories to maintain a healthy weight, and you need protein to help rebuild tissues damaged by the anticancer drugs. You certainly need stamina and as much energy as you can muster to get through the coming months. A well-fed body fights infection more efficiently and, some researchers say, possibly even lessens the severity of some side effects.

As we discuss in Chapter 10, you may have perfectly good reasons for not wanting to eat. Some days, you just may be too tired. People suffering from depression often lose interest in food. And if nausea is troubling you or you have mouth sores, you likely won't want to eat. Ask your doctor for help with these problems, most of which can be fixed.

Mistrusting your sense of taste

One problem that is difficult to fix is your sense of taste. Chemotherapy alters the taste of some foods. You will know right away which foods they are, and it's likely that some of them will be your favorites. Most people report that some foods taste metallic and some taste bitter. Some even taste bland.

Though we generally caution against eating spicy foods during chemotherapy, these foods may taste more flavorful than ever. If you like spicy foods, if they don't bother your stomach, and if you have no mouth or throat sores, go ahead and enjoy a curried dish or something with jalapenos now and then.

Here are some other ways to add flavor to your food:

✔ Marinate meat, poultry, or fish in fruit juice, wine, or a favorite salad dressing before cooking.

✔ Make good use of seasonings, such as basil, thyme, oregano, and rosemary.

✔ Garnish foods with oranges, and, unless you have mouth sores, eat the garnish.

✔ Cook your vegetables with onion, bacon, or bits of ham.

Boosting your appetite

If you and your doctor have fixed what you can and made peace with what you can't, perhaps you can resolve any additional appetite problems by making a solemn vow to eat better every day during chemotherapy treatments. Then throw out all the rules you've ever followed about what, when, and where you had to eat. If you can't locate your appetite, try some of the following tricks and see if it shows up:

✔ **Eat six meals a day.** Nobody says they have to be large meals. But six times a day, sit down to a small meal or hearty snack. As you eat, remind yourself what a big favor you are doing for your body.

✔ **Eat with others.** Family members and friends may choose not to join you for all five or six of your meals, but whenever possible sit at the table — at home or at a favorite restaurant — with people who care about you. As you pass the time talking and laughing, you may find yourself eating more than you had planned.

✔ **Clean your plate.** But do so only if you want to, because you can always save some for later.

✔ **Become a snacker.** Fill individual plastic bags with a selection of snacks you enjoy — think raw baby carrots, sesame sticks, strips of fresh red bell pepper, pistachio nuts, graham crackers, or dried apricots. If you're heading out in the yard to pass some time relaxing in a lawn chair or you hear your recliner in the den calling your name, grab a bag and have a snack.

- ✔ **Try new foods.** Ever eat a mango? Have you tried jicama? Wonder what chicken tetrazzini tastes like? Don't be shy. If a neighbor or friend drops by with a dish you have never heard of, dig in.

- ✔ **Try a different chair.** If you always eat in the kitchen, move to the dining room. If you usually sit at the dining room table, spread a cloth on the coffee table and enjoy the view of the living room as you dine. Maybe your mother never let you watch television while you ate dinner. Now you can.

- ✔ **Drink up.** If solid foods simply do not appeal on a given day, supplement your diet with beverages. Soups, chili, and vegetable juices all count as food, and sometimes they go down more easily when served in a coffee mug. Also, don't overlook liquid nutritional supplements.

Cutting back on drinking

Alcoholic beverages do not count as food. You may find that a small glass of wine or a few sips of beer may stimulate your appetite, but keep in mind that alcohol interferes with some anticancer drugs. Also, it's a bad idea to mix alcohol with the anti-nausea medicine that you may take right after treatment. Check with your doctor before you indulge.

Troubleshooting Skin and Nail Problems

Skin problems associated with chemotherapy — and there are about half a dozen — range from serious to annoying. Let's start with the most serious one first.

Some anticancer drugs delivered through an IV literally can burn your skin and cause permanent tissue damage if the drugs leak out of the vein. Chemo nurses, of course, know to watch for this when setting you up for treatment, but any time you feel a burning sensation when you're getting IV drugs, speak up immediately.

Other anticancer drugs given through an IV may cause skin along the vein to darken. You can wear long sleeves to conceal the discoloration, which fades considerably after treatments end.

If you suddenly develop a severely itchy rash or hives, your skin could be telling you that you're having an allergic reaction to a medication, a bug bite, or some unknown cause. Call your doctor and report the circumstances immediately, as you may need special treatment.

Other, mostly minor, skin problems that you may encounter during chemotherapy include

- Dryness
- Itching
- Peeling
- Redness
- Acne

Because you may have experienced some of these skin conditions even before you were diagnosed with cancer, you likely have some idea how to cope with them and care for yourself. But when skin problems plague you during cancer treatments, they seem to take on an extra urgency, as they represent one more thing on a long list that you have to deal with. Following are some suggestions for dealing with these irritations.

Itching to scratch

Dry, Itchy, and Peeling may sound like an upstart law firm, but it actually sums up the likely state of your skin during chemotherapy. One woman we know insisted throughout her treatments that her face felt like sharkskin, which is said to be so rough that one touch can cut a person. We don't think anyone who touched her face was injured in any way, but still, changes in your skin texture can be upsetting. Here are some ways to alleviate discomfort, both physical and emotional:

- **Moisturize incessantly.** Buy whatever lotion or cream suits you (or is on sale), and apply it often to your dry, itchy skin. Cow's udder balm (really!) and lotions with vitamin E are particularly soothing. The most important time to apply lotion is just after you step out of the shower or bath. Don't dry off, and don't stand around long enough to air dry. Grab that bottle of lotion and moisturize!

- **Take short showers or baths.** Speaking of the shower or bath, long soaks and hot water both contribute to dryness. During chemotherapy, make sure the water is never hotter than warm, and remember to pop in, wash up, and get back out quickly.

- **Use mild skin products.** Find a moisturizing soap that appeals to you, and put your harsh deodorant soap away for now. Also, perfume, cologne, facial toner, and aftershave lotion that contain alcohol all will dry your skin.

> ✔ **Invest in specialized products.** You may want to consider buying a container of pure talcum powder or baby powder and using it as dusting powder. (Stay away from cornstarch — it may promote fungal infections or retard healing.) Also, some people like colloid oatmeal baths, which can help relieve itchy skin.

Knowing how to treat nails

Your nails may give your skin some competition when it comes to crying out for help. Nails may turn dark, become brittle, or crack, or you may notice vertical lines or bands on them. A nail strengthener may help, but it may also cause further irritation.

If your cuticles become red, swollen, or painful, you may have developed an infection and need antibiotics. Call your doctor and report any of these symptoms immediately.

To protect your nails from cuts or possible infections, wear gloves when washing dishes, gardening, or working around the house. If your nails become excessively dry, ask at your local nail salon about an oil product or moisturizing cream made especially for nails.

If the idea appeals to you, slather lotion onto your nails and hands just before bed and sleep in soft, white cotton gloves. Doing so prevents the lotion from rubbing off before it has a chance to sink in, and you should wake the next day with softer hands. And if your feet are extra dry, grease them up with petroleum jelly and wear socks to bed.

Attacking acne

When you are a teenager, acne seems like a tragedy. When you are an adult, acne seems positively insulting. And yet, acne is one possible side effect of chemotherapy. If your face breaks out, make a point to wash your face often with a gentle cleanser and dry it carefully. Ask your doctor or chemo nurse to recommend a mild medicated cream to treat the acne.

Suffering from sunburn

While undergoing chemotherapy, you may find that your skin is more sensitive to the sun. You will know right away, of course, if your skin turns redder than normal after just a short period of exposure to the sun.

Rethinking makeup

Typically, foundation makeup is available for oily, normal, and dry skin. No matter what you had before, it's a good bet that now you will need to head for the products displayed for dry skin. Even so, your skin may refuse to absorb some liquid foundations, and pressed or loose powder may just sit there on your face, mocking any of your efforts to present a nice appearance.

Take time to visit a cosmetics counter at a department store near you and calmly explain your situation. The sales clerk may have advice about foundation and facial moisturizers, as well as tips to help you draw on eyebrows that match one another. (If a near match is the best you can do — and that's quite possible — we think that's good enough. Few people have truly symmetrical features naturally.)

Another option is to ask if your medical center sponsors workshops presented by a representative from "Look Good, Feel Better," a national public service program founded in 1989 to help women with their makeup and wigs while going through chemotherapy (visit www.lookgood feelbetter.org).

An ounce of prevention is in order here: Before you go out in the sun, ask your doctor or chemo nurse whether your anticancer drugs will make your skin more sensitive to the sun. If so, ask them to recommend a sun block that won't irritate your skin. Another solution is to avoid direct sunlight as often as possible. You may even want to wear long-sleeved shirts, long pants, and a hat when you go out.

Reacting to radiation

Here's another reason your oh-so-sensitive skin may turn red: If you had radiation treatments before chemotherapy, or if you are having both treatments at the same time, you may develop *radiation recall.* This condition occurs when the skin where you were treated with radiation turns red — anywhere from light to significantly bright — and the skin may itch or burn for hours or even days.

Be sure to tell your doctor if this happens in case there are specific measures that your doctor wants you to take. In the meantime, about all you can do to relieve radiation recall is to place a cool, wet cloth over the reddened skin. And keep in mind that skin that has been radiated must always be protected from the sun's rays.

Part IV

Radiation: What to Expect and How to Deal with Side Effects

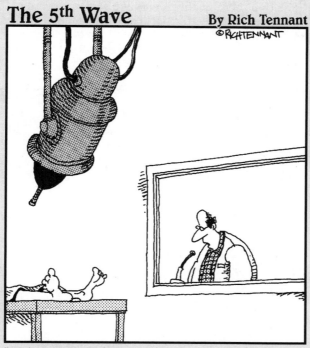

The 5th Wave   By Rich Tennant
©RICHTENNANT

"We're almost finished with your radiation treatment, Mr. Denton. Just lie still and move the Cup-A-Soup a little to your right."

In this part . . .

Radiation therapy only *seems* like something out of science fiction — this part explains exactly how it works. You also find practical suggestions to help you cope with side effects, including tips for caring for your skin throughout treatments.

Chapter 12

What to Expect During Radiation: Tattoos and Moisturizer

*R*adiation zaps cancer cells. If you're a science fiction fan, you may have thoughts of the nifty laser guns that aliens and space warriors use. Outwardly, a radiation treatment isn't as dramatic as a space battle fought with laser guns, but the outcome still can be spectacular.

Here's a sneak peek at what happens during a radiation treatment: The room is dark, and you lie perfectly still on a cold, hard table. No one else is in the room, but if you speak, the technical specialist in charge of your treatment responds immediately. A beam of high-energy radiation is aimed at the site of your tumor — that beam's job is to disable the cancer cells by damaging their DNA structure and "repair system," which prohibits them from continuing to divide and multiply.

Over time, the cancer cells die. The body goes to work breaking down the dead cells, moving them through the blood to be excreted. Some healthy cells also are disabled by radiation. Some recover quickly, beginning repair work within hours after a treatment. Some healthy cells do not recover, and that's why people undergoing external beam radiation therapy have side effects.

That's the process in a nutshell, but when you're facing the prospect of radiation treatments, you want much more than just a sneak peek. That's why we wrote this chapter. In the pages that follow, we walk you through the radiation process in detail, so you know what to expect during the first appointments and the treatments that follow.

Your First Appointments: Getting the Toughest Ones Out of the Way

Radiation therapy may or may not be the first plan of attack against your cancer. You may walk into your first radiation appointment having already had surgery or chemotherapy, but that's not always the case.

As we explain in Chapter 5, there are two main types of radiation therapy: external beam radiation, also known as *teletherapy,* and internal radiation therapy, or *brachytherapy.* The type most appropriate for you depends on:

- The kind of cancer you have
- The stage or grade of your tumor
- Whether your doctor has recommended surgery in conjunction with other treatments

Sometimes, both kinds of radiation treatments are used together to treat cancer — external beam radiation to destroy cancerous cells in the area surrounding the tumor, and internal radiation therapy to deliver a higher dose of radiation at the exact site of the tumor. Of the two, external beam radiation — which is used to treat cancers of the head and neck area, breast, lung, colon, and prostate — is far more common.

Regardless of whether you've had other cancer treatments prior to starting radiation, and regardless of which type of radiation therapy you're preparing for, you undoubtedly want to know what to expect when you walk through the door for your first appointment. The sections that follow take you through each step of the process.

Knowing what to expect

Radiation treatment centers are usually located within hospitals. Maybe you anticipate that your first appointment will involve a brief tour of the facility and a chance to meet the staff. Maybe you don't have any idea what to expect. If that's the case, we have a surprise for you.

You will actually have two "first appointments" — planning sessions that take place before you ever receive a treatment. Here is the laundry list of what will take place at these two appointments:

✔ You will get a body cast.

✔ You will have a CT scan.

✔ You will practice receiving a treatment.

✔ Your radiation dose will be determined.

✔ Your skin will be marked for treatment.

✔ You will set up your treatment schedule.

Frankly, the first appointment is a snap, and the second isn't really so difficult as it is lengthy. Okay, it's difficult because everything you're doing is a new experience, but armed with the information in this section, you can walk in knowing that all you really need to survive these two setup appointments is a healthy dose of patience. Moreover, you will walk out after that second appointment knowing exactly what to expect from a real radiation treatment.

Mapping the area to be treated

Think of your radiation oncologist as a seamstress: Before she can sew anything, she needs to design a pattern to follow. Before your doctor can design a therapeutic treatment for you, you must cooperate to help create a specific plan that targets the cancer cells and protects as many healthy cells as possible. Putting together this plan is a complex process. You're involved, but mostly in the way that a dressmaker's form patiently stands by while the seamstress does most of the work.

In radiation therapy, the treatment field is called a *map*. The map ensures that the radiation is delivered to the right location on the body when treatments begin. Mapping is a two-step process. Before your radiation oncologist can create the map, you must first have a body cast made especially for you.

Creating a body cast

Every day throughout your radiation treatment (which will probably last six weeks or more), you have to lie still on a treatment table in exactly the same spot each time. A personalized body cast — made of Styrofoam plastic and a foaming agent — helps make it easier for you to do so comfortably.

The soft Styrofoam pellets and the foaming agent come in a kit. During your first appointment, the technologist mixes up the ingredients in a thick plastic bag and places the bag inside a wooden structure. You lie down on top of the bag. Once mixed, the ingredients generate a bit of heat, and the bag molds itself to the shape of your body. Within 10 to 15 minutes, the plastic hardens, retaining your body shape.

Getting a CT scan

Also during your first appointment, as you lie in your newly created body cast on the treatment table, you will have a computer-assisted tomography (CT) scan. This is a completely painless test where you lie on a table for about 15 minutes as a scanner moves over your body. The details revealed in the cross-section images from such a scan help determine the treatment field, or map, for your radiation therapy. (Later, during your treatments, a repeat CT scan can help determine whether the tumor is responding to treatment.)

Your radiation oncologist and a physicist or dosimetrist (whose roles we explain in Chapter 5) use the CT images to come up with a map, or pattern, for your treatment — a process that takes 48 to 72 hours. When the map is ready, you will be asked to come back for a simulation session. This session, which may take an hour or so, provides an opportunity for your doctor to try out the map.

Simulating a treatment

At the simulation session, you will be asked to hop up on that cold, hard treatment table once again. Your cast will be put in place, and you will be asked — expected, actually — to lie perfectly still. (You may want to bring headphones and listen to some of your favorite music during the process. Ask your doctor if that would interfere in any way, but it likely won't.)

You will see a machine called a *simulator* that stands in for the actual treatment machine, which is known as a *linear accelerator*. Think of the simulator as an x-ray machine that rotates around you as you lie on the table. As you lie there, your doctor and the other staff will take x-rays and measurements to ensure that the map, or treatment field, is accurate. They will make any necessary adjustments.

During the simulation, feel free to speak up if your leg falls asleep or your arm aches from holding still. The simulation sometimes takes an hour or so, and your doctor and the technicians may be able to alleviate some discomfort if you speak up.

Here are some tips for staying calm while you're on the table:

- ✔ Remind yourself that this is part of a necessary process.
- ✔ Take a few deep breaths as you stretch out.

- ✔ Consider going on a mental vacation — maybe to the beach or the mountains.
- ✔ Expect to be moved a bit this way or that, several times.
- ✔ When you are moved, quickly return to "dressmaker's form" mode and go back on vacation.

Determining the dose to use

At the simulation session, your radiation oncologist and a team of technicians determine the right dose of radiation for you — a dose that delivers the maximum amount required to damage and kill cancer cells while minimally affecting healthy cells. Factors that determine what dose is right for you include

- ✔ The size of the tumor
- ✔ The extent of the tumor
- ✔ The type of the tumor
- ✔ The grade or stage of the tumor

For more information about types of tumors, see Chapter 2. To read more about stages and grades of tumors, see Chapter 3.

It's normal to worry about being dosed with radiation. Just remember that the dose will be carefully calibrated exclusively for you. Be sure to ask any questions you may have about what is planned for you.

During the simulation session, your doctor will probably remind you that radiation passes through the cancer cells and exits your body. In other words, you are not radioactive after a treatment session. You don't glow in the dark, and you aren't capable of grilling meat by pointing your radiated body part at a slab of ribs or a choice cut of sirloin.

Getting tattoos

After you've been mapped, the technician will tell you that now you are ready to have the map marked on your skin. The markings — dark lines or dots that outline the treatment field and need to stay on your skin for the duration of your treatment — can be done with a Sharpie marking pen or with tattoos. Whether you're a fan of body art or not isn't really important.

These days, most medical centers use Sharpies, touching up the lines on a weekly basis so that they won't fade away. At the end of the treatments, the marks are gently "erased" with an ink removal product.

Radiation tattoos are created using India ink. Here's what the tattooing process entails: A technician pricks you with a sharp needle between four and eight times, leaving small, dark blue dots about the size of freckles near the tumor site. These tattoos are permanent, but they are tiny and hardly noticeable.

Does the tattooing process hurt? A little less than a flu shot and a lot less than getting an ear pierced. Any discomfort you feel is brief.

Setting up your schedule

Before you leave your second appointment, you set up your treatment schedule. Though the simulation session takes a while, when you begin reporting for the actual treatments, you'll quickly discover that it takes more time to change out of your street clothes and into your gown than you spend on the table getting your cancer cells zapped.

Radiation treatments generally are given once a day, Monday through Friday, for six weeks or whatever length of time your doctor prescribes. When planning for the daily radiation treatments, figure that you will be at the hospital for 20 to 30 minutes each day.

Usually, hospitals offer treatments between 8 a.m. and 4 p.m., though some stay open until 5 p.m. Why the bankers' hours? Frankly, hospitals are big businesses. The employees may wear white coats or blue scrubs, but the specialty "service departments" are fully staffed only during regular business hours.

Your doctor will explain that to get the best results from radiation therapy, you need to keep every appointment, showing up five days a week for as many weeks as your presence is required. Radiation therapy is a cumulative process — every treatment builds on the last one — so you want to make getting there a priority.

You can (and should) request an appointment time that suits you. Usually, you are expected to arrive at the same time each day, a tactic devised to encourage you to set aside that time each day for a treatment and also to help you remember when to arrive. In that regard, it's no different from adapting your schedule to play tennis every Tuesday morning or bridge every Thursday evening.

You will not feel better or worse depending on the time of day you are treated. If you are working throughout your treatment, you may want to get the appointment over with early, before heading to the office. Or you may want to come in on your lunch hour. Consider what your day ordinarily holds, and make the best choice for you.

Experiencing the Real Thing

You wake up one morning and realize that this day will be different, because this is the day you begin radiation treatments. So much has happened in the short period of time that has brought you to this day. A physical symptom or the result of a blood test raised a warning flag. You were tested further and diagnosed with cancer. Perhaps you've had surgery, and maybe you've been treated with anticancer drugs, either to shrink a tumor or to wipe out any cancer cells remaining in your body.

Since then, you and your doctor have discussed any options you may have regarding your radiation treatment. Together, you have made the best choice, and you have educated yourself about what to expect from the particular type of radiation therapy you'll receive. You have discussed what side effects you may experience and put strategies in place to combat them. (For more on side effects from radiation, see Chapter 13.) And now here it is — the day you will have your first radiation treatment.

Assessing your feelings

How are you supposed to feel about starting radiation?

How you are supposed to feel, of course, doesn't really matter. How you do feel is what counts. You may feel anxious or even scared. That's normal. You may feel eager to get started, to get the first one out of the way, so you can find out for yourself what it's like.

You can take heart in knowing that you are well prepared. After all, you've already survived the first two appointments. Your body cast awaits, your simulation is complete, your tattoos are in place, and your schedule is established. You've been to the medical center. You've met the staff. You've had a tour. You are familiar with a treatment table, and you know what to expect from the linear accelerator. You're mapped, marked, and ready to go!

Arriving on the first day

Your first real appointment may last a little longer than a typical treatment, just because you're new at this. Still, no matter what the day brings, rest assured that you are fully prepared. When you first arrive, the staff will greet you warmly, eager to shepherd you through the steps involved. You will undress and don a gown.

You must not use any moisturizer on or near the area being treated for at least two hours before each daily treatment. Unfortunately, that soothing goo interferes with the treatment. Consider taking a tube of moisturizer with you to the hospital, and get in the habit of slathering up after each appointment. (See the upcoming "Soothing Your Skin" section for more information.)

When it's your turn in the treatment room, technicians will put you in your body cast and then place you in exactly the same position you practiced with the simulator. Your doctor may stop by to check your position, and you may need x-ray films or ultrasound images to further evaluate your position.

Then comes the easiest part of all.

Actual radiation therapy usually lasts only five to ten minutes. You hear some buzzes or clicks from the *linear accelerator* (see Figure 12-1) — the machine delivering the radiation — but you feel nothing.

After the treatment, you return to the dressing room, moisturize the zapped area, dress, and go on your way. That's it!

Your doctor may ask to meet with you once a week for a few minutes after a treatment to examine you. This visit is always a good opportunity to ask more questions or discuss side effects. If you have questions between visits, feel free to call your doctor or speak with the nurse on duty or the radiation oncology staff.

Making good use of your time on the table

Some people meditate during radiation treatments. Some visualize the cancer cells being zapped, crumpling up, and dying. Some concentrate on growing hair that has been lost during chemotherapy. Some make plans for the future. One woman we know always tells people what worked for her when she was going through cancer treatments. "I cast my anchor far into the future," she says. "My husband kept planning exciting trips for me after treatments were over and for years to come. How could I disappoint him?"

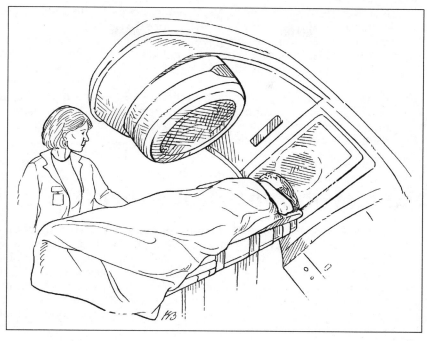

Figure 12-1: A linear accelerator typically is used for external beam radiation.

A note about questions: No question is off limits, and there is no such thing as a silly question. The people providing your radiation treatments have heard it all, and they are eager to educate you, comfort you, and even laugh with you, so speak up!

Soothing Your Skin

External beam radiation treatments may cause your skin to burn, especially if you are being treated for skin cancer, breast cancer, or head and neck cancers. You can help protect your skin even before treatments begin by moisturizing frequently.

In fact, the preparation presents an opportunity for a friend who is looking for a way to help you. Consider asking someone to accompany you to a neighborhood drugstore to stock up on moisturizers. Planning ahead and completing your shopping in advance brings peace of mind and allows you to check that task off your "to do" list.

Not everybody's skin burns. Also, among those who do burn, some burn less than others. However, if you have pale or sensitive skin that you routinely have to protect from ordinary sunlight, you likely will experience some irritation from radiation. (You can find detailed information about side effects from radiation therapy in Chapter 13.)

Extra moisturizing before radiation therapy begins is a good idea, just to give your skin a slight advantage. However, keep in mind that you cannot use any moisturizer on or near the area being treated for at least two hours before each daily radiation treatment.

Making Wardrobe Adjustments

After each radiation treatment, you will want to use moisturizer on the area treated, but you may not want to slather up and put back on your work clothes. If you are being treated for skin cancer, breast cancer, or head and neck cancers, you may want to plan ahead for any wardrobe adjustments you may have to make. Start by thinking about what articles of clothing typically touch the area that will undergo radiation therapy. Plan to temporarily substitute soft, well-washed fabrics for the clothing that now touches that body part.

Specifically, if you are being treated for breast cancer after a lumpectomy, you can expect the radiated breast to swell and be especially sensitive to the touch. You may want to stock up on larger bras, and you'll want them in soft cotton, if possible. Another option is to buy men's white T-shirts, wash them to remove any sizing sprays or other fabric coatings, and wear one in place of a bra. The shirt will help protect your skin and keep moisturizing lotions off your outer clothing.

Also, although people generally associate hair loss with chemotherapy, radiation treatments can cause hair loss if the head is being treated. If you are a female, investing in a wig or several scarves before treatments begin may be a good idea. See Chapter 10 for detailed information about dealing with hair loss.

Seeking the Support You Need

In Chapter 8, we offer specific suggestions for ways to get help and support from your spouse, your children, and your friends — all of whom are probably eager to help make your life easier during your cancer treatments. We encourage you to take a close look at the information in that chapter.

On taking sandwiches

Author Wendy Reid Crisp tells a great story in her book *Do As I Say, Not As I Did* (Perigee Books) that clearly illustrates the arts of giving and receiving.

Several years ago, her hometown had three devastating earthquakes within 18 hours. Much of the town fell down. Wendy's friend Pam called to say that another friend's house had collapsed.

Nancy, the woman who lost the house, went with Pam to the Red Cross station at the local fairgrounds to see what they could do to help.

Once there, Pam suddenly said, "Nancy, take a sandwich. We're the victims here. We don't always have to be the ones who make the sandwiches. Sometimes, we have to be the ones to take the sandwiches."

Make lists of various tasks (such as driving you to radiation appointments and helping you with grocery shopping) that your loved ones can assist with, and don't hesitate to delegate them. Doing so not only frees up some of your time and energy so you can focus more fully on getting healthy, but it offers the people close to you constructive outlets for their emotions regarding your cancer.

You need to do everything possible to take care of yourself during the many weeks that you'll be going through radiation therapy. And your family and friends want to help take care of you, too. Even if you're not used to being on the receiving end of such generosity, try to graciously accept what is offered, as that will be a great gift for everyone.

Giving Yourself a Break

We've said this before and we'll say it again — everything changes when you are diagnosed with cancer. Of course, many of the changes in your routine at home and at work are temporary, in place only for that period of time necessary while going through your treatments. Peace with these changes comes as you adapt to the new "normal," as you grow to trust your doctors, and as you refine your strategy for success (which we discuss in Part V of this book). Along the way, make it easy on yourself. Cut yourself some slack whenever possible.

As a wise woman once advised during a life-disrupting situation of a different sort, "If you find you can't live up to the high standards you have set for yourself — well, you'll just have to lower them."

Keeping your appointments

While looking for ways to give yourself a break, you may zero in on that unwieldy daily schedule of radiation treatments. You may go so far as to consider skipping a couple of treatments. Maybe you have a project due at work, and leaving early on Tuesday is inconvenient. Maybe you promised the kids you would take them to see a movie on Friday afternoon. Maybe the mere idea of being at the same place at the same time, day after day, goes against the grain of your free-spirited self.

Think again. Radiation therapy treatments are scheduled every day, five days a week, for six or more weeks, for a reason.

Research shows that external beam radiation therapy is most effective when given continuously. The daily zap causes more damage to the cancer cells than a random zap now and then, and the intensity of the schedule also allows cancer cells less time to repair themselves.

Lots of studies have reported the same finding. One study at Istanbul University in Turkey reviewed records of 853 women, ages 21 to 87, who had received radiation therapy after breast cancer surgery between 1990 and 1999. Researchers compared survival rates for women who stopped their radiation therapy for more than a week with women who had no interruptions in their radiation treatment.

Radiation therapy worked for both groups, but the women who did not interrupt treatment had higher overall survival rates after five years and also after ten years, and their recurrence rate also was lower. Based on the study, the researchers reported that interrupting radiation treatments for eight days or more may make radiation therapy less effective in women after breast cancer surgery.

Keeping everything in perspective

Now you know why it's important to make time every day for your radiation therapy for the entire course of treatment. That said, if an ice storm blows into your city and keeps you from the hospital for a day or two, don't panic. You can make up the time at the end of the schedule with no harm done.

Another short-term interruption in treatment may occur if your doctor advises you to skip a day or two to allow your skin more time to heal. (Read more about that in Chapter 13.) Again, you can make up the days missed at the end of the schedule.

Keeping an eye on the future

Wasn't it Willie Nelson who said "Nothing lasts forever except an old Ford and a natural stone"? No matter.

Radiation treatments, part of a process designed to help you survive cancer, do not last forever. In fact, in the context of your whole life, the six or seven weeks that you must devote to radiation treatments is a very short time. Even when you factor in the hours spent ahead of time worrying about radiation treatments and the time spent afterward as your skin heals, we still are talking about a short period of time.

Earlier in the chapter we mention a woman who said that she cast her anchor "far into the future" even as she did what was necessary day by day during her cancer treatments. Her positive, forward-thinking approach may also work for you.

Chapter 13

Coping with Side Effects of Radiation Therapy

....

In This Chapter

▶ Finding the energy to fight fatigue

▶ Protecting your skin

▶ Dealing with intestinal disarray or lymphedema

▶ Fending off infection

▶ Confronting hair loss

▶ Getting help for depression

....

*A*s a local, or site-specific, treatment for cancer, radiation therapy goes right to the trouble spot, which may be the site of a tumor in need of shrinking or the place where a tumor was surgically removed. Radiation therapy is relentless (in the best sense of the word), returning to the trouble spot again and again, day after day, week after week, zapping that tumor or any lingering cancer cells with vigor and purpose until the job is complete.

During this relentless zapping, some healthy cells are damaged. Sometimes, the delivery system is to blame for side effects. Sometimes, the destruction of healthy cells keeps your body from functioning normally, and that leads to side effects. Either way, the focused approach of radiation therapy means that most side effects occur only at the site being treated. Notice the word *most,* because some side effects do express themselves elsewhere. The side effects can be uncomfortable, but all of them can be addressed.

One unanticipated side effect may be more trips to the service station, resulting in higher gas bills. Most people undergoing external radiation treatments must show up at the hospital or treatment center five days a week for anywhere from one to eight weeks, depending on the type of cancer, the location of the cancer, the type of equipment used at your radiation oncology center, and other related circumstances. The rigorous schedule may lead to frustration and impatience because sometimes during radiation, time seems to crawl. On the other hand, the daily treatments may help you become more patient — a one-size-fits-all virtue that you will find handy in other situations as well.

Patient or otherwise, in this chapter you find information on such side effects as fatigue, skin problems, inflamed mucous membranes, intestinal disarray, lymphedema, pneumonitis, urinary irritations, a drop in white blood cell count, hair loss, and depression.

If you are undergoing chemotherapy as well as radiation and you have read Chapters 9, 10, and 11 on possible side effects of chemotherapy, some of the material in this chapter will sound familiar. That's because some of the side effects are the same, though they don't always manifest in the same way. However, if you are being treated only with radiation, you won't need to refer back to the chapters on chemotherapy — much of what you want to know about side effects is right here, and additional information is in Chapter 15.

Considering What's to Come

No one likes to think of herself or himself as "most people," yet you may take heart knowing that most people report no significant side effects from radiation therapy. Some report a few side effects, and only a handful of individuals encounter a host of difficulties. Generally speaking, any side effects you may experience won't begin until after the second or third week of treatment, and most will fade away (literally and figuratively) several weeks after your final treatment.

After radiation therapy is complete, almost all side effects go away. With any luck, the only reminder of your treatment will be any permanent radiation tattoos (which we explain in Chapter 12).

You may have heard that radiation therapy can cause cancer in the course of treating that very disease. In Chapter 5, we explain that radiation has been used to cure cancer for more than 100 years. This is not a new technology. However, it is an ever-evolving technology, and the science is better than ever. At this point in time, the benefits of radiation therapy far outweigh the tiny risk of developing additional cancer.

The risk of developing cancer while undergoing radiation treatments is very small. What is much more likely to happen is that radiation therapy will cure or control the cancer you already have.

Identifying your type of therapy

As we explain in Chapter 5, there are two main types of radiation therapy: external beam radiation, also known as *teletherapy,* and internal radiation therapy, or *brachytherapy.* The type of radiation therapy your doctor(s) will recommend for you depends on these factors:

- ✔ The kind of cancer you have

- ✔ The stage or grade of your tumor

- ✔ The site to be treated

- ✔ The prescribed dose

- ✔ Whether you are undergoing chemotherapy at the same time

- ✔ Whether your doctor has recommended surgery in conjunction with other treatments

- ✔ Whether you have an underlying medical condition that may make radiation therapy hazardous to you

- ✔ The technical expertise and particular experience of your radiation oncologist, and the equipment and staff with which she works

Sometimes, both kinds of radiation treatments are used together to treat cancer — external beam radiation to destroy cancerous cells in the area surrounding the tumor, and brachytherapy to deliver a higher dose of radiation at the exact site of the tumor. That said, external beam radiation — used to treat cancers of the head and neck area, breast, lung, colon, and prostate — is the more common of the two.

Predicting your experience

Most people report no significant side effects from radiation therapy. Those who do usually experience them after the second or third week of treatment.

Because everyone responds to cancer treatments differently, we can't say exactly what, if any, side effects you may experience. More than likely, your body's reaction to radiation treatments will depend on the following:

- ✔ The type of cancer you have

- ✔ The location of the cancer

- ✔ The stage and grade of cancer

✔ Your general health

✔ Your age

✔ Whether you have fair skin (which is more likely to burn) or darker skin

We can say that one of the most important things you can do while undergoing treatments is to drink a lot of water. Staying well hydrated may help you fend off some of the side effects or lessen their impact. If we had to predict one single side effect that you would be most likely to experience, it would be fatigue, so that's where we'll start.

Fending Off Fatigue

General fatigue is the side effect that people undergoing radiation therapy most often report. Unlike the fatigue that chemotherapy causes, the fatigue that radiation treatments often bring is not severe. Most of the time, you will easily be able to go about your daily routine with just a few adjustments to the schedule. In the later weeks of radiation therapy, one adjustment that may help considerably is to schedule a nap, maybe late in the afternoon before dinner. Sometimes, just cutting back a bit on normal activities or going to bed an hour earlier makes all the difference.

Learning an important word

In Chapter 10, we make a recommendation regarding our favorite way for people going through chemotherapy to save energy. This recommendation may come in handy for you during radiation treatments as well. Basically, we encourage you to learn to say "no." The word "no" is especially important as you learn what you can and can't do during treatments and how to find the balance in between.

Let's practice. Face yourself in the mirror and repeat saying "no" until it loses all power to make you feel guilty, ashamed, or somehow less than you are.

"No" is a perfectly legitimate word and an exceptionally powerful tool if you truly want to conserve your energy. When you are tired, use this word whenever you or anyone else asks you to do anything that can be put off until later, anything that really doesn't have to be done ever, anything that someone else could easily do for you, or anything that you sense will send you over the edge into total exhaustion.

Saying "no" to someone else often is a way of saying "yes" to yourself.

Getting your timing right

Here are some additional tips that will serve you well as you safeguard the energy you do have:

✔ **Pace yourself.** If you are working full-time or even part-time while undergoing radiation therapy, you know you need to give much of your energy to your employer. Still, save some back so you will be able to enjoy family activities and time spent with friends. If you know you will be busy Thursday night, plan to take it easy on Wednesday evening. If Sunday is a big day for you, lie low on Saturday. Take into account on a day-to-day basis how much energy you have and divide it up accordingly. That two-letter word comes in handy here.

✔ **Change your pace.** Some days, your energy may last well into the evening before fatigue sets in. Some days, you'll be ready to call it quits by midafternoon. And some days, morning will come and you will have nothing to offer the day in terms of energy. Change your pace accordingly. A famous 12-step program advises taking it one day at a time. When you're being treated for cancer, feel free to take it a half day at a time. If that's the best you can do, that's more than sufficient.

✔ **Plan your day.** Each morning, write down or make a mental list of what you hope to accomplish in the course of the day. You should know right away if you are expecting too much of yourself. If so, reassign some tasks to another day or — even better — to another person.

✔ **Include naps or breaks in your plan.** No plan is complete without one or more opportunities for short naps or breaks on those days when your energy runs low. Stretch out on the couch or lean back in an easy chair to rest your eyes for a minute. If you slip into a full-fledged nap that lasts 20 to 30 minutes, so much the better.

✔ **Schedule a day of rest.** After an unusually busy day that can't be avoided, schedule a relaxing day for yourself.

✔ **Get a little exercise.** Research has shown that even a short walk can help decrease fatigue. You may think that exercise will make you even more tired. You may be right. On the other hand, just a little exercise each day may bring you some renewed energy.

✔ **Fuel the body.** Even when your health is at its peak, your body requires fuel to function efficiently. Be sure you eat a nutritious diet during radiation therapy. (For more information, see Chapter 15.) Protein and carbohydrates, particularly, provide essential fuels.

✔ **Consider complementary therapies.** Some people find that fatigue decreases if they practice guided meditation or guided imagery or spend some time in prayer. (See Chapters 14 and 16 for more on these therapies.)

Caring for Your Skin

External beam radiation treatments may cause your skin to burn, especially if you are being treated for skin cancer, breast cancer, or head and neck cancers. The fairer your skin, the more likely it is to burn. Darker skin tends to *bronze,* or take on the appearance of a deep suntan. In both cases, the skin becomes dry and more sensitive. In Chapter 12, we recommend that you begin to moisturize your skin even before treatments start, to give your skin an extra advantage.

Your skin works hard to resist entry to anything introduced from an outside source. In fact, moisturizers don't really add moisture to the skin, but they help keep moisture from escaping out of the skin by closing all the exits.

Moisturizing works best when the skin itself is wet. If you are so inclined, soak your radiated part from time to time in a lukewarm bath devoid of fragrant bath gels or bubbles. When you leave the bath, reach for your favorite moisturizer and apply it to your damp skin.

Using protective strategies

Here are some tips for protecting radiated skin:

- Avoid applying heating pads or ice packs to your skin.
- Protect your skin from harsh deodorants, deodorant soaps, heavy perfume, and clothing made of rough cloth.
- Expose the radiated area to open air whenever possible.
- After a bath, dry your skin carefully, patting it with a fluffy towel.
- Avoid exposing radiated skin to direct sunlight.

Watching for warning signs

As we discuss in Chapter 12, some people may experience an excessive skin reaction during radiation treatment. The signs of this reaction include

- Dramatic darkening
- Peeling

   ✔ Itching

   ✔ Excessive tenderness

   ✔ Blistering

   ✔ Ulceration of the skin

If your skin shows any of these reactions to radiation, tell your doctor immediately. You may need to use an antibiotic cream or cortisone ointment until your skin heals.

Soothing Inflamed Mucous Membranes

The moist layer of tissue that lines body cavities such as the mouth, nostrils, throat, and bowel are called *mucous membranes*. Radiation therapy can interfere with these mucous membranes, causing inflammation and irritation. If your head or neck is being treated, you may develop a sore throat, mouth dryness, a cough, or hoarseness. If you are having radiation therapy for lung cancer, the mucous membrane of your *esophagus* (the tube that food goes down when you swallow) may become extremely irritated. Here are some ways to cope with these symptoms:

   ✔ Eat soft foods — think soups, milkshakes, and ice cream.

   ✔ Drink plenty of fluids.

   ✔ Suck on hard candies or lemon drops to help produce saliva.

   ✔ Ask your doctor about a tablet that stimulates the salivary glands and minimizes mouth dryness.

   ✔ Ask your doctor about cough suppressants, analgesics, or steroids to reduce the inflammation and irritation.

Experiencing Diarrhea

If you receive radiation to the pelvis, stomach, abdomen, or bowel, you may experience diarrhea. Your doctor can recommend several different drugs to help alleviate it.

Don't let diarrhea trouble you more than 24 hours without calling your doctor. You don't want to risk dehydration.

More than likely, you experienced diarrhea at some point before you were diagnosed with cancer, so you probably already have some ideas on how to control it and help care for yourself at the same time. Here are some tips:

- **Drink, drink, drink.** Mild, clear liquids are best — think water, broth, ginger ale, or a sports drink — served at room temperature. If you're drinking ginger ale or a citrus-flavored soft drink, pour it in a glass and wait until the drink goes flat.

- **Eat small meals throughout the day.** Low-fiber foods are best, including white rice, noodles, mashed or baked potatoes, fish, and skinless chicken or turkey. Stay away from high-fiber foods such as whole grain breads, cereal, beans, nuts, seeds, popcorn, raw vegetables, and any kind of fresh or dried fruit. Lay off milk products for now as well.

- **Take in some potassium.** You lose potassium when you have diarrhea, so help to replace it by eating bananas, oranges, and potatoes. Peach and apricot nectars both are good sources of potassium, too, so if you find them appealing, drink up.

Saying "No" to Nausea

Nausea is a possible side effect if you receive radiation treatments to the pelvis, stomach, or abdomen. Usually, if this side effect is going to trouble you at all, nausea sets in about two hours after a treatment. If that happens, your doctor can recommend several drugs to help alleviate the problem.

Don't let nausea trouble you more than 24 hours without calling your doctor, because you run the risk of dehydration.

Making wise food choices

More than likely, you experienced nausea on occasion even before you were diagnosed with cancer, so you probably already have some ideas on how to control it and help care for yourself at the same time. If you are troubled by nausea, here are some practical suggestions that may help you feel better:

- **Eat before you get up in the morning.** Try a couple of crackers or some dry cereal so you have something in your stomach before you start your day. You can put the crackers on a bedside table each night before you go to bed.

↙ **Avoid spicy foods.** Tacos, curries, and pepper steak come to mind. Other no-no's include greasy foods and any foods with strong odors that may unsettle your stomach. One way to avoid cooking odors, of course, is to eat only cold foods.

↙ **Eat several small meals.** Spreading your meals throughout the day ensures that you never have an empty stomach. Also, chew your food thoroughly.

↙ **Take in some protein.** Get the biggest bang for your buck by eating such foods as eggs, tuna, or peanut butter. If these foods seem to upset your stomach, stick to high-carbohydrate foods such as rice, pasta, or potatoes.

↙ **Stay away from sweets.** The rich desserts, doughnuts, and Danish rolls will have to wait.

Making wise drink choices

Ironically, both dehydration and over-hydration can induce nausea, so you want to balance the amount of fluid in your stomach at any one time. Here are some tips:

↙ **Sip small amounts.** It may take conscious effort at first, but you need to learn not to swallow too much at a time.

↙ **Drink from a straw.** That's one way to insure that you don't drink too much.

↙ **Drink only liquids at room temperature.** Beverages that are too hot or too cold may upset your stomach.

↙ **Drink before and after meals instead of while you eat.** If you feel at all woozy, you don't want to send down too much at one time.

↙ **Stick to unsweetened fruit juices.** Clear juices, such as apple, are best.

↙ **Defizz carbonated drinks.** Try a few sips of a clear carbonated beverage, such as ginger ale, that has been allowed to go flat.

↙ **Settle in with a cup of tea.** Remember to drink it warm, not hot. Peppermint tea is known for soothing the stomach.

↙ **Avoid caffeinated drinks.** Caffeine may make you feel worse.

Finding comfort

Even when you don't feel good, comforting yourself can improve the situation. Here are some strategies:

- **Remove tight clothing.** This is the time to wrap yourself in an old, cozy bathrobe or climb into your favorite stretched-out sweats.

- **Take deep, slow breaths.** Concentrate on your breathing to keep it even, and try to relax any tight muscles, especially in your stomach.

- **Strap on a wristband.** People worried about seasickness on cruises wear wristbands that touch acupressure points. You can find these wristbands at your local pharmacy.

- **Suck on ice chips.** Or, if you prefer to suck on hard candy, try peppermint or lemon drops.

- **Put a cold cloth over your eyes.** Try lying down for 30 minutes (unless you've just eaten).

- **Get plenty of rest.** If you can relax enough to have a nap, you likely will feel better when you wake up.

Living with Lymphedema

Radiation therapy occasionally can result in *secondary* or *acquired lymphedema,* which is an accumulation of lymphatic fluid that leads to swelling of the arms or legs. When radiation therapy damages healthy lymph nodes and vessels, scar tissue forms that interrupts the normal flow of the lymphatic fluid through the body. Another possibility during radiation treatment is that burned or blistered skin can lead to lymphedema.

Continual moisturizing of dry or burned skin can keep blisters from developing and cut down on the risk of lymphedema.

The earlier that lymphedema is diagnosed and treated, the better the outcome. If you do develop lymphedema, several treatments are available, including

- Manual lymphatic drainage (a gentle form of massage)
- Bandaging
- Changes in skin care and diet

✔ Compression garments (sleeves or stockings)

✔ Exercises

If any given body part receiving radiation treatment begins to swell, speak with your doctor. If redness, warmth, or tenderness develops, you may have an infection. Here is the Catch-22: Extremities with lymphedema are more vulnerable to infection, and an infection may result in lymphedema. Avoid infections whenever possible (see the upcoming section "Watching Your White Blood Count" for advice), and if you get one, get it treated right away.

Looking Out for Pneumonitis

Sometimes, radiation therapy can cause *pneumonitis,* or inflammation of the lung tissue. If you are being treated for lung cancer, your doctor will take special precautions when setting up the map, or pattern, for your treatment. In Chapter 12, we explain that the map ensures that the radiation will be delivered to the right location on the body. With three-dimensional conformal radiation therapy, your radiation oncologist can decrease the amount of healthy lung tissue affected by treatments, but he can't avoid it altogether.

Three-dimensional conformal radiation therapy (*aka* 3D-CRT) calls on computers and computer-assisted tomography scans (*aka* CT or CAT scans), along with magnetic resonance imaging scans (*aka* MR or MRI scans), to create a three-dimensional representation of a tumor and the surrounding organs. Tools called *multileaf collimators,* or *blocks,* match the radiation beams to the size and shape of the tumor. This allows for less radiation exposure to nearby normal tissue.

If you're going to get pneumonitis, generally it starts about 30 days after your radiation treatments end and may last up to three months. Symptoms include a dry cough and shortness of breath when you exert yourself, and these are symptoms you want to report to your doctor. Usually, the inflammation goes away on its own and no medication is required, but if it lingers, your doctor may prescribe low-dose steroids.

Running to the Restroom

Sometimes when the bladder or *urethra* (the tube that carries urine from the bladder to be excreted) is radiated, you may notice an increased need to urinate or some irritation while urinating — the same symptoms that a mild bladder infection brings. These symptoms are temporary, and your doctor may recommend a urinary analgesic and advise you to drink plenty of fluids. Water is the beverage of choice.

Beverages with caffeine — coffee, tea, cola, and some other soft drinks — may make these symptoms worse.

Watching Your White Blood Count

A small percentage of people undergoing radiation treatments develop a depressed white blood count. That may happen if your bone marrow, lymphocytes in your blood stream, and lymph nodes are exposed to radiation during treatment. Generally, the drop in white blood cells is temporary, but if a simple blood test reveals that your white blood count is low enough to cause concern, your doctor may want to stop treatments for a few days to allow the count to go back up.

In Chapter 2, we explain how white blood cells help protect you from infection. Doctors have different strategies to boost production of white blood cells, though these strategies are rarely needed during radiation therapy.

If you want to help in your body's effort to protect you from infection, you can take some simple precautions:

✔ **Avoid sick people.** These days, many people show up at the office sick when they should have stayed home in bed. If at all possible, don't share the morning paper, the boss's report, or a bag of chips with anyone at work who has a cold or infection. At home, resist snuggling with any member of the family who is ill.

✔ **Wash your hands.** Visit the sink often, not just before and after eating or after using the toilet. Use lots of soap and warm water. Lather up good, and go to it.

✔ **Avoid cuts and bruises.** Germs hang out in cuts, and this is no time to have to do battle with germs. If you do get a cut or a wound, clean the area well with soap and water. If the cut is shallow, consider pouring hydrogen peroxide over it for extra protection, and then put on a sterile bandage. If the cut is deep, call your doctor.

If you are a knife-wielding home cook subject to the occasional accidental cut, consider buying a steel mesh kitchen glove or cut-resistant glove to protect yourself. Kitchenware shops and home goods departments in some stores carry the gloves for about $15.

✔ **Stay out of crowds.** Who knows what germs may lurk in the bodies of fans gathered at a football game, shoppers filling up the mall, or enthusiasts flocking to a music concert? We're not saying you can't have any fun. Just have fun with smaller groups of people right now. And if ever there was a time to learn to love shopping online, this is it. Yes, you have to pay for shipping, but consider that cost the price of safeguarding your health.

✔ **Eat only cooked food.** Raw fish, raw seafood, raw meat, and raw eggs all may serve as a haven for bacteria. When your immune system is functioning normally, you're not likely to be bothered by this bacteria. During cancer treatments, the bacteria in uncooked food could represent a threat to your health.

✔ **Reassign pet cleanup tasks.** Pet waste — from dogs, cats, birds, and reptiles — is another source of bacteria. If you must be the person responsible for cleaning up after a family pet, wear rubber gloves. After the deed is done, wash the gloves. Then, just to be sure, wash your hands.

Dealing with Hair Loss

Radiation therapy causes hair loss only in the area being treated. For instance, if your lower body is being treated, you likely will lose pubic hair or leg hair. If your chest or a breast is undergoing radiation, hair on and under your arms will come out. If your head or neck is being treated, you likely will lose scalp hair, and you may also lose your eyebrows and eyelashes.

Depending on the type of radiation and the dose, hair loss that results from radiation may be permanent. Often, the hair cannot grow back because the hair follicles are damaged too severely.

Check with your radiation oncologist so you know exactly what to expect regarding hair loss. You may not suffer much when your doctor tells you that your leg hair won't come back or the hair under one arm will never grow again. Hearing that you will be bald from now on may be a lot harder. If your hair is going to come out, expect to lose it about two or three weeks after treatments begin.

Pampering your hair while you have it

While you still have hair, you want to treat it well. Here are some tips that will help keep your hair — and your scalp — healthy when you begin radiation treatments:

✔ Invest in a mild shampoo.

✔ Brush your hair with soft strokes using a soft hairbrush.

✔ Refrain from dying, perming, or relaxing your hair.

✔ Put away the brush rollers.

✔ Use only the low setting on your hair dryer.

✔ Protect your scalp from the sun.

Even before you lose any hair, your skin will be more sensitive during radiation therapy.

Making plans in advance

Because hair loss is such an emotional experience (for men as well as women), spend some time getting used to the idea of yourself without hair, especially if your doctor expects the loss to be permanent. The idea is to figure out how to maintain a positive body image after your hair is gone. For obvious reasons, this is easier to do before you lose your hair.

Choosing a wig

If you are a woman, think about whether you will want a wig. If you want a wig and you think you will prefer to recognize yourself in the mirror, visit a wig shop before your hair falls out so you can match your current style and color. You may think that visiting the wig shop will be a grim expedition. It doesn't have to be. We recommend that you take a friend who makes you laugh, and then go out for lunch afterward. You may even decide to try a wig that is a totally new style and color of hair for you. If price is not an issue, get two!

Most insurance companies pay for one wig — which they call a *prosthesis* — for people undergoing radiation therapy. If your insurance company will not pay for a wig or you don't have insurance, contact your local branch of the American Cancer Society. Women who have recovered from cancer often donate their wigs and other head coverings, and these are available for free. Also, some medical centers have a wig "exchange" where you can find an attractive covering for your head.

Wigs can be made from human hair (which is very expensive) or from synthetic hair (which is much more reasonably priced). All wigs, even expensive ones, require some care. For tips, see Chapter 10.

Sometimes, wigs cause a rash on the scalp, especially in summer when your scalp perspires under the wig. The best way to treat this rash is to expose your bald head to the open air as often as possible. Rub on a mild, over-the-counter cortisone cream if needed. If that doesn't work, by all means speak with your doctor. When you want to wear the wig, place a piece of clean

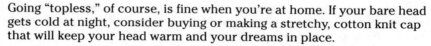

cotton fabric between your scalp and your wig — an old, well-washed bandanna, folded to fit, is perfect. It won't show, and the cotton will absorb the moisture that caused the rash.

Choosing an alternative head covering

A wig is not your only option:

- ✔ Some women prefer to wear a scarf or turban instead of a wig after they lose their hair.

- ✔ Most men — and a few women — go about with bald pate gleaming. Will people stare? Some may; if they do, just flash a confident smile and go on your way.

   Going "topless," of course, is fine when you're at home. If your bare head gets cold at night, consider buying or making a stretchy, cotton knit cap that will keep your head warm and your dreams in place.

- ✔ Some people invest in a signature hat to wear outdoors to protect their bald scalps from sunburn, which is important all the time but especially so during cancer treatments.

All these decisions are personal, so do whatever feels right for you. There are no rules except those you make, and you can always change the rules to suit yourself.

Cutting your hair

You may want to make an appointment to have your hair cut short. This proactive approach provides you with an emotional way station between having a full head of hair and none at all. If all your hair comes out, it's easier to manage losing short hair than long — for a while, anyway. And if only a little of your hair ends up falling out, the hair that is left will look thicker and fuller if it's short.

Hair falls out in single strands and in clumps. Once it starts coming out, hair will lie on your pillow, litter your collar, and coat the walls of your shower. Frankly, it's a mess — such a mess that you may find yourself dialing your hair stylist and asking for an appointment to have your head shaved.

If you suspect that you may become weepy while having your head shaved, ask if you can schedule the appointment after hours or if there is a private room where you can get the job done and then don your wig or head covering before leaving the salon. Keep in mind that you are not the first person to make this type of call, and you will not be the last. Most stylists are happy to do what they can to help you through this difficult appointment.

Replacing eyebrows and lashes

Whether to replace your eyebrows and lashes is a personal decision: Some women choose not to bother, and some feel comforted when they look in the mirror and see the eyebrows and lashes they expect to see.

If you are a woman accustomed to running an eyebrow pencil over your brows to thicken or darken them, you may do fine when it comes time to draw them on from scratch. If you've never owned an eyebrow pencil, you may want to buy one before treatment begins and pay attention to that bony arch above each eye. That's where the brow goes. Usually, a natural brow starts out fairly thick near the bridge of the nose, thickens slightly right above the iris, and then tapers off on the other side. You can actually buy a set of eyebrow stencils and play around, seeing what shape suits you. Some people opt for permanent cosmetics, or tattooed eyebrows. If that interests you, make an appointment before your eyelashes fall out so the aesthetician can match the color and shape of your natural brows.

As for eyelashes, you could invest in a pair of false eyelashes or glue on false lashes one at a time, though that strikes us as a lot of trouble. You could also put a little eyeliner on the edge of each upper and lower lid. Another option is tattooed eyeliner, which you would have forever.

"Look Good, Feel Better" (www.lookgoodfeelbetter.org) is a national public service program founded in 1989 to help women with their makeup and wigs while going through cancer treatments. Many hospitals present workshops conducted by representatives of this program.

If your medical center does not have such a program and you want help drawing on eyebrows or putting on makeup, stride boldly into a nearby department store and ask one of the makeup consultants at the cosmetics counter to help you. This service is free.

Recognizing Depression

Not all side effects are physical. Being diagnosed with cancer can cause emotional pain and even extreme anxiety and depression. You may worry how you got cancer and how you will cope with the diagnosis and treatment. You most assuredly will worry — or at least wonder with great intensity — whether your treatments will be successful and you will survive.

Asking for help

If you have a case of the blues, first try to elevate your own mood or seek out a support group. (See Chapter 17 for some suggestions on how to choose such a group.) If you think your blues have reached a point where you need professional help, speak with your doctor. Some symptoms of depression that indicate a call for help include

- Withdrawal from other people
- Decreased appetite
- Heightened sense of anger
- Feelings of hopelessness
- Uneven sleep patterns
- Lack of personal hygiene
- Loss of any pleasure in pleasurable activities

Don't wait for someone else to make the first move. No one knows better than you how you feel and how you are coping emotionally with cancer treatments. Help is readily available; if you need it, do yourself a favor and speak up.

Your doctor can recommend trained counseling professionals who can help you cope with your feelings. Among the options are

- Psychiatrists
- Psychologists
- Social workers
- Clergy
- Counselors trained especially to work with people going through cancer treatments

If necessary, your doctor (or a psychiatrist) may recommend medications to help lift depression. If you do decide to take medication, talk with your radiation oncologist first to make sure that the drug will not interfere with your treatments.

Working through fear and grief

The moment when you fully realize that you may not live forever, as you (and the rest of us) had planned — when you realize that indeed cancer may carry you off long before you are prepared to go — is a difficult moment. Faced with that moment, many people find themselves mentally zipping through several of the well-documented stages of grief. Those stages are

- Denial
- Anger

- ✔ Bargaining
- ✔ Despair
- ✔ Acceptance

What causes this fear to abate? The passing of time and the end of treatments, at least when the cancer is curable. Fear also subsides when you have the surprising — and somewhat embarrassing — revelation that people with cancer are not the only people left in the dark on this very personal and important matter. No one gets a guarantee. Really, all you can do from this moment on is vow to live now and to live better.

Part V
Your Success Strategies: Assembling Your Support Team

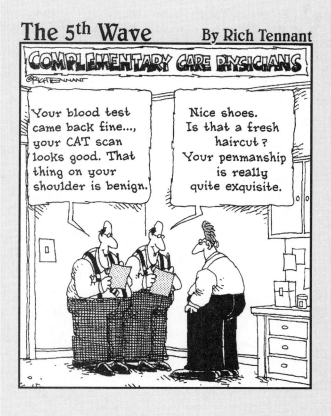

In this part . . .

No one goes through cancer alone. Starting with getting the most out of your appointments with your doctor, this part gives you tips on assembling a support team of healthcare professionals and others to help you get through the good and not-so-good days.

Chapter 14

Your Health Professionals: Your Friends and Guides

. . . .

In This Chapter

▶ Maximizing your relationship with your doctors

▶ Making a bad situation better

▶ Sounding out a psychologist

▶ Assembling a personal team of health professionals

▶ Finding classes and workshops on complementary therapies

▶ Sampling six practices that may enhance your quality of life

. . . .

*E*ven when the prognosis is good and your doctors predict the best possible outcome, living with the burden of a cancer diagnosis is difficult. During treatment, regardless of the prognosis, you're likely to spend time worrying how you will cope with surgery, whether the treatments are working, how you will handle any side effects, if you will be able to do your job, how your family will fare when you're not at you're best, and whether your insurance company — if you are fortunate enough to have insurance — will pay most of the bills or refuse to cover tests and procedures that your doctors recommend.

Frankly, juggling these concerns would wear out a healthy person, and just now, your health is compromised. Sometimes, it may be all you can do to get through the day.

The best way to lighten the burden is to divide it. Remember the African proverb that says it takes a village to raise a child? You may not need an entire village to get you through cancer treatments, but assembling a team of health professionals to help you will make this difficult time easier.

The best place to start, assuming family and friends are already on board, is with your doctors: the medical oncologist, surgeon, radiation oncologist, and your family doctor or internist. In this chapter, we provide ideas to help you successfully share responsibility for your care with your doctors. We also explain the benefits of seeing a psychologist. And we suggest ways to build useful relationships with massage therapists, yoga teachers, reiki practitioners, tai chi instructors, masters of meditation, and fitness experts. All these individuals can be helpful members of your support team.

Go team!

Communicating with Your Doctors

Ideally, you have chosen your doctors carefully, you trust them, and you already enjoy a relationship that allows you to be open, to ask anything on your mind, and to get thoughtful responses in return. You also will be pleased to know that all your doctors will speak with one another on a regular basis throughout your treatment, sharing test results and reports on your progress, in order to maintain a coordinated approach to your care.

You and your doctors will be seeing a lot of one another, and as your treatment progresses and you get to know each other better, your confidence in each other is likely to grow.

Building a good relationship

You can begin building a good relationship with your surgeon, medical oncologist, and radiation oncologist by asking questions about your treatment and by speaking up about your concerns and fears.

Maybe you're the type of person who wants to know everything there is to know at your first appointment. That, of course, may not be possible — although we do know of one doctor who will not leave the treatment room during a first appointment until a patient says she has no more questions. Some of this doctor's initial appointments are lengthy, but because he previously has extended the same courtesy to everyone sitting out in the waiting room, returning patients do not complain.

Assuming that you can't learn everything you want to know the first time you speak to your doctor, you want to make good use of future appointments. Following are some tips on how to do that.

Jotting down questions

After your first appointment — no matter how long it lasts — just about the time that you reach the parking lot, you likely will find yourself with a head full of questions. You already know by now that the idea of having cancer is hard to absorb, plus all the information about treatments and side effects is brand new.

You may want to buy a small spiral notebook in which to write questions that occur to you in between appointments. If a question is urgent or your health is in danger, absolutely pick up the phone and call your doctor's office. Otherwise, make a note of what you want to ask, and take the notebook with you to your next appointment.

What kinds of questions will you likely want to ask? Here are some suggestions:

- ✔ How long will it take to recover from any surgery I may have?

- ✔ How can I expect to feel during treatment?

- ✔ What are the possible side effects?

- ✔ What treatments are available for the possible side effects?

- ✔ How can we make it easier for me to get through treatments?

- ✔ Are any clinical trials available that are testing innovative new treatments for my cancer?

- ✔ Do you have colleagues I should consider seeing if I'd like to get a second opinion?

You should also ask any questions you have about information on cancer treatments that you've heard on television or read on the Internet. At this point, almost every doctor has had more than one patient come in clutching a 26-page printout from one or more Web sites, with pertinent sections underlined in red or highlighted in yellow. These printouts give your doctor an opportunity to respond in a number of ways, including

- ✔ Cautioning you against believing everything you read

- ✔ Going through the printouts with you to address areas of concern

- ✔ Providing you with additional printed materials from other sources or recommending reliable medical sites on the Web

- ✔ Gently (or otherwise) suggesting that you confine your reading about cancer to topics that specifically affect you

> ✔ Referring you to a Cancer Information Center where trained personnel can help you separate the reliable information from unreliable information

Asking questions is a healthy sign that you are involved in your care and working with your doctor toward the best possible outcome from your treatment. Most doctors welcome questions. If your doctor does not, or if she seems threatened by your questions, you have every right to ask why. You are, after all, a person — not simply a disease waiting in line for treatment to be issued, or a room number on the oncology floor of a hospital — and you just happen to be affected by a potentially life-threatening condition.

Taking notes

So say you bought a spiral notebook to jot down your questions in between appointments. Consider flipping it over. Beginning with the last page, work your way in toward the center, using this section of your notebook to write down what your doctor says in response to your questions. Recording the answers will be helpful for a number of reasons:

> ✔ You won't have to count on your memory.
>
> ✔ You can review the written answers to your questions as many times as you need to.
>
> ✔ You can remind the doctor about a particular question and answer later, as your treatment progresses, and ask if the same answer still holds true.

You also may use this side of the notebook to record any new instructions or suggestions. If you find that you are too upset or distracted to make notes during appointments, ask a friend to come with you and take over that task.

You may want to ask the doctor whether she would object if you tape-recorded important conversations, so you wouldn't need to take notes.

Speaking frankly

Truthfully, there isn't anything you can say that will shock or unduly upset your doctors. They have heard it all and likely will be eager to either put your mind at rest or assure you that solutions exist for the problems you anticipate. Of course, some of your questions may not be specifically about your treatment but about your concerns or fears. Talk away!

If you have a large number of questions, you may wish to provide them to your doctor in advance of your visit. That way, when you meet for your appointment, he can provide thoughtful, complete answers in an organized fashion and budget the time of your visit in a way that enables your most important concerns to be addressed.

Few of us, thankfully, have previously been in a situation where we had to ask a virtual stranger whether we will die from cancer. If that is the most important question on your mind, speak up.

Maybe your spouse or your parents can guess what's on your mind, but your doctors cannot. If you tell them, they can help. If you keep silent, they cannot.

Don't worry that you may tear up or even sob openly when you ask. That box of tissues on the doctor's desk is proof that this topic has come up before in this room. Of course, some doctors may hedge on the answer, because no one can predict precisely how any one individual will respond to cancer treatments. On the other hand, think how good you will feel if, after taking everything into consideration, your doctor tells you that you can expect to enjoy a feisty old age.

Considering less-than-ideal situations

Unfortunately, not everyone is in an ideal situation when it comes to building good relationships with doctors. For instance, you may experience one of these situations:

- ✔ Your insurance coverage limits your choice of doctors.
- ✔ You live in a small town with a shortage of oncologists or surgeons.
- ✔ Your medical oncologist strikes you as gruff, unresponsive, or unsympathetic.
- ✔ You've heard stories that lead you to mistrust the surgeon.
- ✔ Something about your doctor or the office staff just rubs you the wrong way.

If any of these examples rings true for you, you may want to investigate changing doctors, even if your choices are limited. If that's not possible, you may have to change your attitude and make the best of the situation.

Enjoying a good relationship with someone responsible for your medical care during cancer treatments is important and a worthy goal. No one is saying that you and your doctor must have dinner or plan a fishing trip together! But, as adults, most of us understand that even a poor relationship can be made better when both parties acknowledge that they are working toward the same goal.

On the other hand, maybe the problem is not with the doctor. Perhaps these factors are part of the equation:

- ✔ By nature you are introverted.
- ✔ In general, you are reluctant to express personal thoughts.
- ✔ Maybe you have trouble thinking of yourself as a healthcare consumer and feel more comfortable taking a passive role in your treatment.
- ✔ Perhaps you remain so overwhelmed or fearful regarding your diagnosis that you simply are unable to move forward.

The benefits of working to build a good relationship with your doctors are many, among them the reassurance that you do not have to face cancer alone, which is no small matter. When you talk frankly with your doctor and establish open communication, you share the burden of your cancer diagnosis and gain a clearer understanding of how your doctors and your medical treatments can help you.

That said, we know that some people feel that the relationship with their doctors and upfront advocacy for themselves are not as important as getting the right treatment from qualified individuals. It's your call.

We encourage you to quickly resolve problems that exist in your relationship with your doctors or to make peace with these problems, and then start concentrating on getting through treatments.

Seeking Help from a Psychologist

Typically, cancer and fear walk hand in hand. You may as well invite fear in to sit down at the table with you so you can form an alliance with one another. We're not saying this will be an easy alliance, but confronting your fears puts you in a position to determine which are real and which are imagined, and then you can rank them according to priority. At that point, you will know whether you can dissolve your top-rated fears or whether you must acknowledge them, and then you can move on with your life.

Fear of death is a biggie, but it is not the only fear that people face after a cancer diagnosis. Additional fears among people undergoing treatments for cancer, described in 1994 by researchers Irene Pollin, a social worker, and Susan Golant, a medical writer, include

- ✔ Fear of loss of control or helplessness
- ✔ Fear of loss of self-image (feeling less attractive, physically weaker, or somehow damaged)

 ✔ Fear of a stigma and feelings of shame

 ✔ Fear of abandonment

 ✔ Fear of expressing anger

 ✔ Fear of isolation (physical, social, and emotional)

Certainly, your doctors can help alleviate these fears and others that may arise during treatment. Doctors also are accustomed to hearing angry outbursts from time to time from people frustrated with their treatments, their diagnosis, or even their fear. If fear or anger takes hold and prohibits you from living any semblance of a normal life while undergoing treatments, your doctors may recommend that you meet with a psychologist.

Such a recommendation is not a cop-out and does not represent any sort of dereliction of duty. Your doctors, after all, are primarily concerned with your medical care, and they need the time they spend with you to address medical concerns, present medical information, and answer your medical questions. That level of responsibility can be overwhelming when you consider that insurance companies, hospital leadership, and practice administrators routinely pressure doctors to see more patients in the course of each day.

Don't be insulted or feel put off if your doctor recommends that you see a person who specializes in emotional well-being.

Allowing yourself to accept help

In some segments of society, even today, seeing a psychologist carries a stigma. This is unfortunate.

You get to decide whether you will try to get help or whether you will allow what other people may think to keep you from getting it.

If you do decide to meet with a psychologist, consider asking your doctor to recommend two or three names. Check with your insurance company to make sure treatment is covered, or call to find out if any of the psychologists recommended offer a sliding fee scale. You may want to schedule introductory meetings with these individuals to determine which of them makes you feel most comfortable.

In spite of what you may have seen in movies, seeing a psychologist does not require that you lie on a couch and explore childhood traumas. Instead, you likely will find yourself sitting in a chair across from a kindly person who is eager to help you cope better with the changes that cancer has brought into your life.

Knowing what kind of help to expect

What, exactly, can a psychologist do to help? A number of things, including teach you practical skills to help you cope better as you go through treatments. These skills, if you practice them faithfully, may help you to

- Reduce fear and anger
- Eliminate or alleviate depression
- Deal with questions about fertility or sexuality
- Encourage emotionally healthy behaviors
- Communicate better with your family, your friends, and your doctors
- Limit emotional responses to side effects
- Improve your general quality of life

Meeting Other Health Professionals

At some point in your treatment, a member of your medical care team may recommend that you explore other resources to increase your overall sense of well-being. If your doctors neglect to make this recommendation, feel free to ask if they have any objection to your adding other health practitioners to your support team. These individuals may include

- Massage therapists
- Yoga teachers
- Reiki practitioners
- Tai chi instructors
- Meditation instructors
- Fitness experts

We fill you in here on each of these complementary therapies. Notice that we do not refer to these practices as *alternative* therapies. Sometimes, the two words are used interchangeably, but they have two different meanings. People sometimes seek out *complementary* therapies, such as yoga or reiki, while undergoing chemotherapy or radiation therapy. *Alternative* therapies, some of which claim to cure cancer, are used in place of a chemotherapy regimen or a course of radiation treatments.

Of the alternative therapies that have been scientifically tested, some have been found to be ineffective or even dangerous. Clinical trials have revealed that a few alternative therapies have produced results that warrant further study, but to date the Food and Drug Administration has not approved any of them for public use.

The time-tested complementary practices included here are considered just that — methods of self-care that complement traditional medical care — and they are in no way recommended to take the place of traditional care. Just to be safe, check with your doctor before making an appointment or signing up for a class.

You don't need to take up all the practices we discuss in this chapter, but you may want to make room in your life to benefit from one or two. If you are interested in finding someone in any of these fields who works in your area, here are some suggestions:

- ✔ Ask if your hospital or medical center offers the service you want.
- ✔ Call your local community center or YMCA to ask about classes.
- ✔ Explore adult education programs offered through school districts and colleges in your area.
- ✔ Do an Internet search — type in the pertinent word and the name of your city and state.
- ✔ Consult your Yellow Pages.

Making time for massage

Uptight? Tense? Tired all the time? That sounds about right! Licensed massage therapists will tell you that a good massage relaxes you and increases your energy. Other benefits to stretching out on the table (see Figure 14-1) include

- ✔ Stress reduction
- ✔ Improved circulation
- ✔ Shorter recovery time for strains or sprains
- ✔ Enhanced flexibility

Remain unconvinced?

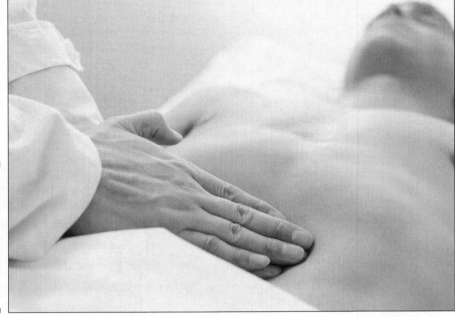

Figure 14-1:
A thera-
peutic
massage
may help
ease
anxiety,
fatigue, and
pain.

Source: © Getty Images/Ryan McVay

A recent study conducted by Memorial Sloan-Kettering Cancer Center in New York reveals that "a relaxing session with a certified massage therapist appears to help reduce anxiety, pain, fatigue and other types of discomfort in cancer patients." There's more — the study also reported that most patients "still feel better two days after the massage."

Drs. Barrie R. Cassileth and Andrew J. Vickers, authors of the study, reported their findings in the *Journal of Pain and Symptom Management* in the fall of 2004. For the study, the authors talked with 1,290 cancer patients who had signed up for a therapeutic massage. They asked the individuals to rate their physical discomfort before and immediately after massage, and again two days later. Participants reported that massage reduced their symptoms of fatigue and discomfort by about 50 percent.

Oncologists estimate that about one in five cancer patients in the United States have therapeutic massages in the course of treatments. If you are interested in having a therapeutic massage, seek out a certified, licensed therapist. (Certification and licensing requirements vary from state to state.) Tell the therapist you are undergoing treatments for cancer and that you may need a lighter touch than someone who is not. Typically, people having therapeutic massage undress fully for the treatment. Though much of your body is covered with a sheet or blanket throughout the massage, if you prefer to leave on your underwear, tell the therapist that as well.

Many hospitals and medical centers now have licensed massage therapists on staff and offer outpatient appointments in a special wing or quiet area where massages take place. Generally, the rates are as much as $15 lower than those at a health spa or fitness center.

How frequently will you want to schedule a massage? That depends on several factors. The budget matters, of course. On the other hand, you may feel so much better after a massage that you will be inclined to find the money once a month. Otherwise, massage therapists recommend that you periodically monitor whether you are breathing freely and fully and making the most of your energy. In other words, let your body tell you when you need a massage.

Yearning for yoga

Maybe you've tried traditional hatha yoga, the physical discipline of developing control of the body through asanas or poses. Maybe you have expanded your repertoire and attended hot yoga classes, in rooms heated to 90 degrees or more, or taken up one of the many other styles of yoga. Or maybe you know little about it or think the only people who practice yoga are strict vegetarians.

Surprise! Yoga classes, now available in every nook and cranny of the country, are filled with office workers and laborers, college students and older adults, the physically fit and those in search of the same. Yoga classes also are offered for pregnant women, children, and people in prison.

A short history of yoga

Yoga developed in India as a system within the Hindu religion more than 5,000 years ago. The word *yoga* comes from the Sanskrit root *yuj,* which means "to yoke," "to unite," or "to be whole." The ultimate goal of each of the many styles of yoga is the balance of body, mind, and spirit. Some people say they are interested only in the physical aspects of yoga, so some yoga teachers choose not to discuss the spiritual aspects of the practice. Others portray yoga as a "mental practice," as well as a physical practice. Vicki Lander, a yoga instructor we know in St. Louis, notes that "all your senses are turned inward" when practicing yoga, "and that is the opposite of how we are the rest of the time."

Some forms of yoga are too demanding for someone going through cancer treatments. However, one practice, called *restorative yoga,* is ideal. In a restorative yoga class, you spend the entire time on a mat on the floor. You take just a few poses, compared to more active classes, and you use blankets, bolsters, and blocks to help support your body as you gently stretch (see Figure 14-2). The emphasis here is on relaxation through measured breathing, and the goal of restorative yoga is to reduce stress and restore energy.

No less an august body than the National Institutes of Health has announced that "yoga may also be an appropriate way to relieve symptoms, such as fatigue and nausea, associated with cancer and treatment." Accordingly, since 2000, the Cancer Supportive Care Program at the Stanford University Medical Center in Palo Alto, California, has offered free restorative yoga classes to help cancer patients deal with "stress, fatigue and symptom management."

If a yoga studio near you offers restorative yoga classes, who can you expect to see in such a class? People in need of some quiet time in the company of others who honor the body's need for deep relaxation. That is why the class is ideal for anyone fatigued from chemotherapy or radiation treatments.

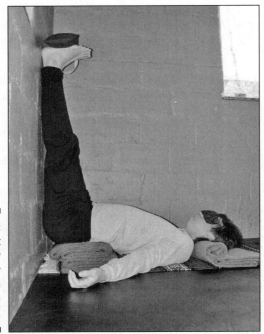

Figure 14-2:
Every part of the body is fully supported in restorative yoga poses.

Source: Wain Winborne/Big Bend Yoga Center

You may not get the maximum benefit from a restorative yoga class the first time or two. If you hang in there, you will learn practical techniques to help you achieve deep relaxation. Eventually, if you choose, you may do the poses at home.

If there is no restorative yoga class where you live, consider heading to a library or local bookstore to look for Judith Lasater's *Relax and Renew: Restful Yoga for Stressful Times* (Rodmell Press). Lasater has taught yoga since 1971. She is a physical therapist and holds a doctorate in East–West philosophy. The book was not written specifically for people going through cancer treatments, but much of Lasater's wisdom is applicable.

Renewing with reiki

Reiki (pronounced *ray-kee*), like massage therapy, is a form of body work, but in this one, you leave on all your clothes and a trained practitioner touches your body lightly. A Japanese word, *reiki* means "universal life energy" and refers to the common energy found in all life. Here is how the Reiki Healing Arts Center in Seattle describes it: "Physicists and mystics alike know that energy is the common denominator in all matter. The Usui System of Reiki teaches us to direct loving energy through our hands to rebalance the natural energy state of all that we touch."

The American Cancer Society's "Guide to Complementary and Alternative Methods" notes that reiki is "a form of hands-on treatment used to manipulate energy fields within and around the body (believed to influence a person's physical and spiritual health) in order to liberate the body's natural healing powers." In other words, by unblocking the body's energy paths, practitioners say they can promote better health.

Among the benefits are

- Lower levels of pain
- Less muscle tension
- Faster healing of injuries
- Improved sleep
- A decrease in stress and anxiety
- An enhanced sense of well-being

Reiki practitioners also say they can help people undergoing cancer treatments. Currently, no scientific evidence exists to support these claims, but some doctors do suggest that reiki may help reduce stress and enhance quality of life for people being treated for cancer. The American Cancer Society reports that "some patients undergoing chemotherapy have reported reduced intensity and frequency of nausea and vomiting after reiki sessions." Also, a small pilot study found that "reiki treatment effectively relieved pain in 20 volunteers, some of whom had cancer."

How does it work?

You climb fully clothed onto a traditional massage table and lie back with your eyes closed. Placing his or her hands on different parts of your body, the practitioner balances the energy within your body and in fields around it. A session lasts between 60 and 90 minutes, and the cost varies, depending on the practitioner. The number of visits required to help any one individual also varies.

Some reiki practitioners also are massage therapists, and some are not. Training programs and certification are readily available, though no government agency regulates the programs.

Reiki is a safe form of body work. But, as always, consult with your doctor before beginning treatments.

When you shop for a reiki practitioner, you may hear instructors describe their training at certain "levels," and you may also hear the term *reiki master.* This term usually refers to someone trained in all levels of reiki who also lives according to the five precepts of reiki. They are

- ✔ Just for today, do not worry.
- ✔ Just for today, do not anger.
- ✔ Earn your living honestly.
- ✔ Honor your parents, teachers, and elders.
- ✔ Show gratitude to every living thing.

As you can see, reiki is a peaceful tradition, and a practitioner just may be able to bring some peace to you as you undergo treatments for cancer.

Taking up tai chi

Tai chi (pronounced *tie-chee*) is an ancient Chinese practice that cultivates and circulates energy throughout the body. Unlike with reiki, no practitioner is involved and no one touches you. Instead, you work with an instructor, moving through a series of sustained, flowing movements (see Figure 14-3) that proponents say balance your energy level internally — which makes you feel better and allows you to do what you need to do. Some people consider tai chi a form of "moving meditation."

Tai chi classes are easy to find; your medical center may even sponsor them. The prestigious M.D. Anderson Cancer Center at the University of Texas in Houston offers tai chi as one of 75 different programs at its complementary therapy center called the "Place . . . *of wellness.*" Why? Its Web site (www.md anderson.org) explains: "At M.D. Anderson, we realize that physical healing is only part of the puzzle. Place . . . *of wellness* is an environment where all persons touched by cancer may enhance their quality of life through programs that complement medical care and focus on the mind, body and spirit." Most of the programs are free, and others cost a small fee.

What does tai chi have to offer a person going though cancer treatments? Clinical trials have shown the potential benefits to include

- ✔ Reduced stress
- ✔ An enhanced sense of well-being
- ✔ Increased balance
- ✔ Improved strength and toning
- ✔ Lower blood pressure
- ✔ Better bone density

"Tai chi teaches us to slow down," says Sue Schulte, an instructor in St. Louis. That's probably because the slow, deliberate movements (called *forms*) each contain between 20 to 100 moves and take as long as 20 minutes to complete. The forms all have names that come from nature, such as *Passing Clouds.* Every movement is practiced on both sides of the body. No particular level of body strength is required to do tai chi.

For best results, proponents recommend spending time doing tai chi each day. After you have taken a class or two and learned some of the forms, you may want to practice at home.

Trying meditation

If you know anything about meditation, you may already know there are numerous methods, including Healing Buddha meditation, the relaxation response, Christian meditation, mindfulness meditation, and many others. Perhaps the best known is Transcendental Meditation. All methods emphasize the benefits of sitting quietly and resting your mind.

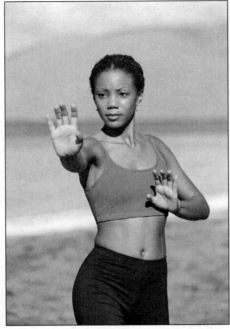

Figure 14-3:
The slow pace of tai chi may add to your energy, rather than increase fatigue.

Source: © Getty Images/Thinkstock

If you don't know anything about meditation, you may think that taking time to sit still in a chair each day sounds silly.

Think again.

An independent panel convened by the National Institutes of Health has approved meditation as "a useful complementary therapy for treating chronic pain and insomnia," and the American Cancer Society suggests that meditation "can help to improve the quality of life for people with cancer." Late in 2003, meditation made the cover of *Time* magazine. Inside, the article stated that scientific research conducted over the past 30 years shows that meditation has much going for it. Among the benefits are

✔ Decreased stress

✔ A reduction in the risk of heart attack and hypertension

✔ The reversal of hardening of the arteries

✔ Increased energy

Furthermore, after you have read a book or taken a class on meditation, you can do it in the privacy of your own home on your own schedule. If you prefer to learn online, the Meditation Society of America, located in Wagontown, Pennsylvania, sponsors the Meditation Station at www.meditationsociety. com. The Web site includes a meditation specifically for people undergoing cancer treatments.

Maharishi Mahesh Yogi developed Transcendental Meditation (TM) more than 40 years ago, based on ancient Hindu principles. Some 5 million people around the world are said to practice TM.

Proponents claim that TM raises your energy level the first time you try it, and they say that it takes only one week to learn the method. After that, you need 20 minutes of quiet time twice a day. If TM interests you, you will be happy to hear that an introductory lecture usually is offered free. See www. tm.org for information on where lectures take place.

Fitting in fitness

Fitness? Isn't it enough that I have cancer and have to go through all these tiring treatments?

If that's what you are asking yourself, just give us time to explain. Some 300 exercise programs are available nationwide for people with cancer. Medical centers sponsor some of the programs, and others are offered at health clubs. Typically, the programs consist of a moderate aerobic workout, stretching, and relaxation exercises. The Cancer Center of Santa Barbara sponsors such a program called "Cancer Well-fit" at the Santa Barbara Athletic Club. Founded in 1994, the supervised exercise program includes

- ✔ Progressive resistance strength training
- ✔ Specialty strength training
- ✔ Group exercise and one-on-one training
- ✔ Mind/body conditioning
- ✔ Aquatic therapy
- ✔ Movement therapy (Pilates, yoga, tai chi)

Classes meet twice a week, and exercises are personalized for each individual according to ability and comfort level. The Cancer Center reports that more than 66 percent of participants consider the program part of their "support network."

Sound more appealing now?

There's more: The University of Minnesota Cancer Center reports that "there is scientific evidence that a program of moderate intensity activity like walking can assist with the symptoms of fatigue often reported by those undergoing cancer treatment." Biking and swimming also are recommended. Talk to your doctor before you begin an exercise program while undergoing treatment.

You don't want to exercise so vigorously that your fatigue level increases. You have to rely on your common sense. If you feel better after you exercise moderately, keep it up. If you don't, cut back until you are stronger.

If exercising is beyond what you are capable of doing right now, consider putting it on your list of things to do later. When you are ready, you can always begin by walking around your block or to the mailbox, and see how you do. If it goes well, try again the next day, and the day after that, and so on. Countless studies conducted in the last 20 years have shown that exercising can enhance your quality of life after cancer.

You may wonder if exercising will prevent a recurrence. Good question. Nobody really knows the answer, though research is in progress.

Some agencies, the American Cancer Society among them, suggest that regular exercise — along with making healthy choices regarding weight, diet, alcohol intake, and smoking — can prevent cancer from occurring in the first place. A study conducted from 1986 to 1999 of 29,564 women indicated that if all the women in the study had followed guidelines for good health issued by the American Institute for Cancer Research, "about 30 percent of their new cancers and cancer deaths could have been prevented or delayed." These guidelines include

- ✔ Not smoking
- ✔ Having a maximum body mass index of 25 and limiting weight gain to 11 pounds after age 18
- ✔ Engaging in daily moderate exercise and weekly vigorous physical activity
- ✔ Eating five or more servings of fruits and vegetables each day
- ✔ Eating seven or more daily portions of complex carbohydrates
- ✔ Limiting alcoholic drinks to one a day (for women)

✔ Restricting red meat to three ounces daily

✔ Limiting fatty foods

✔ Restricting salted foods and use of salt in cooking

To date, research seems to indicate that exercise can reduce the risk of certain kinds of cancer, including

✔ Colon cancer

✔ Breast cancer

✔ Endometrial cancer

✔ Prostate cancer

✔ Testicular cancer

But can exercising prevent recurrence? Again, research continues.

Chapter 15

Good Nutrition: Eating Right No Matter How You Feel

*W*hether you eat to live (with little interest in food or meal preparation) or you live to eat (savoring the aromas, textures, and flavors of well prepared meals), your relationship with food changes during cancer treatments. How? Several ways. For instance, the presence of cancer in your body may cause you to lose interest in food or to become satisfied earlier in each meal, so that you eat less. Radiation therapy can cause a burning, constricting sensation in your esophagus. Chemotherapy can cause foods to taste metallic. Both treatments cause fatigue, meaning that, over time, you may find that you prefer sleeping to eating.

Your preference may have to take a back seat to what's good for you. Good nutrition is always important, of course, but eating right is absolutely crucial during cancer treatments. Think about it. Your body, with the help of your treatments, is fending off further attacks from any cancer. Your body also is busy coping with the many internal changes caused by the treatments. You can help eliminate some additional health problems if you make sure that you eat right.

Think of food as fuel — a continuously renewable source of energy. You know that a car on the verge of running out of gas is unreliable, which means you may not get where you are going in a timely fashion. You also know you will get nowhere fast if the tank is completely empty. So fill 'er up — with premium!

Welcoming New Members to the Team

In Chapter 14, we talk about the importance of assembling a support team, a group of health professionals to help you successfully navigate the time you spend undergoing cancer treatments. If you have nutrition-related problems during treatments, you may have the opportunity to add some additional members to that team:

- ✔ You already have doctors and nurses on the team, and they will help you make certain that you do everything possible to eat right so that you may better tolerate treatments.

- ✔ If you live alone, a hospital social worker may put you in touch with a community program that delivers meals to people who can't cook for themselves.

- ✔ If depression keeps you from eating, a psychologist (see Chapter 14) may be able to help.

- ✔ And you may want to speak with a registered dietitian for specific tips on how to prepare and eat healthy meals during your treatment.

A *registered dietitian* is a trained professional who specializes in food and nutrition. The American Dietetic Association is the professional association for more than 70,000 registered dietitians in the United States. This professional organization sets the standards for all registered dietitians, who work in such diverse locations as hospitals, nursing homes, school districts, health departments, food businesses, and even offices that specialize in sports nutrition. Some registered dietitians have established their own private practices.

Your doctors or nurses may recommend a registered dietitian, or you may find one at www.eatright.org. You simply enter your zip code in the box provided, and names of registered dietitians in practice near you pop right up.

Knowing When You Need Help

Now you know how to find a registered dietitian. But do you know when to make the call? Not to worry. You do not have to make that decision by yourself. Before your treatment begins, your doctors will assess whether you are at risk for nutrition-related problems. At one of your early appointments, you likely will be asked pointed questions, including

- Has your weight changed over the last six months?
- Have your eating habits changed in the last six months?
- Have you experienced any problems with eating recently?
- Are you eating well enough to perform basic daily tasks?

You also will have a physical exam, and your doctor will look for signs of disease, including any loss of weight, fat, and muscle or any fluid buildup in the body. You also will be informed of possible side effects from the treatments and carefully monitored throughout for any signs of nutritional disarray.

Of course, if you experience any side effects or symptoms that affect your eating habits in a negative way, by all means use your mouth for its second-most-important purpose — speak up! Also ask any questions you may have about exactly what to eat and how much of it.

Catching Up on the Food Fights

Not surprisingly, not everyone agrees on what constitutes good nutrition. You probably learned in school about the four basic food groups: dairy, meat, fruits and vegetables, and grains. In 1980, the U.S. government released a guide that expanded on the original four food groups. In 1992, the U.S. Department of Agriculture developed the Food Guide Pyramid, which showcases the foods recommended by that department and the Department of Health and Human Services. In case you have not pulled out your copy of the Food Guide Pyramid any time recently, the guide recommends eating daily servings of various food groups, including bread, cereal, rice, pasta, fruit, vegetables, meat, dairy products, fat, oil, and sweets.

The Department of Agriculture has revised the guidelines every five years since 1980 to reflect new scientific findings. Still, not everyone supports the agency's recommendations. One criticism repeatedly leveled at the Department of Agriculture is that at no time has the size of a "serving" been defined. Other critics say that not all fats are bad and not all complex carbohydrates are good. Some have criticized the emphasis on dairy foods. And still others have protested that not all sources of protein offer the same nutrition.

Personalized pyramids

A nonprofit "food issues" think tank in Boston, known as Oldways Preservation & Exchange Trust, has developed Asian, Mediterranean, Latin American, and vegetarian food pyramids.

In addition to specific food recommendations, these pyramids also call for daily physical activity. To learn more about these pyramids, visit www.oldwayspt.org.

While the organizations involved fight it out, you may want to spend your time finding out about the benefits of good nutrition during cancer treatment, reacquainting yourself with what constitutes "good nutrition," and taking into consideration any particular challenges you may face from side effects as you put together a good eating plan for yourself.

Boning Up on the Benefits

Good nutrition — especially the enthusiastic intake of protein and calories — helps fend off a number of problems. For instance, protein and calories help your body to heal, fight infection, and provide energy. That's why your doctors and nurses are particularly interested in your eating habits at this time. They likely will ask you about them at each appointment — especially if your weight changes — whether or not you bring up the subject.

Sometimes knowing the specific benefits of a particular practice makes it easier to embrace that practice. To that end, the National Cancer Institute has enumerated some of the benefits of eating well during cancer treatments. Good nutrition helps you to do the following:

- Maintain strength and energy
- Protect yourself from infection
- Tolerate treatment better
- Reduce nutrition-related side effects and complications
- Prevent or correct malnutrition
- Prevent wasting of muscle, bone, blood, organs, and other lean body mass
- Recover and heal more efficiently
- Maintain or improve your quality of life

Most likely, these all are benefits you would like to enjoy, so being particular about what you eat just now likely sounds like a good idea. Of course, some nutrients are more important than others. You may want to keep these in mind when putting together a healthy eating plan.

Acknowledging the "A" List

The list of important nutrients to consume during your cancer treatments consists of proteins, carbohydrates, fats, vitamins, and minerals. In the sections that follow, we take a look at each, but first we discuss the most important thing to consume during treatment: fluids.

Finding time for fluids

Staying hydrated is especially important during cancer treatments. Medical oncologists treat a lot more dehydration than malnutrition, so we cannot overstate the importance of drinking.

If you have a choice between eating and drinking, by all means, drink. And first and foremost among recommended fluids is — wait for it — water. Water is cheap. Water is easy to find. Water goes well with both meat and fish. Okay, water goes just fine with any dish at all.

Fruit juices may serve as a secondary source for fluids, followed by milk. Sports drinks have electrolytes, which are particularly important if you are experiencing substantial vomiting or diarrhea. And if your mouth or esophagus is a little sore, try sucking on a Popsicle.

Wondering whether soft drinks are on the list? Yes, but they are at the bottom, along with alcoholic drinks. That's not to say you can't enjoy an occasional soft drink or glass of wine or beer, but these beverages contribute little or nothing to keeping you hydrated.

Pumping up with protein

Regular meals high in protein (see Figure 15-1) can help you maintain nutritional equilibrium during treatments and heal after treatments end. Protein is derived from a variety of foods, including

- Meat
- Eggs

✔ Fish

✔ Poultry

✔ Milk and cheese

✔ Nuts

✔ Beans, peas, and lentils

✔ Soy products

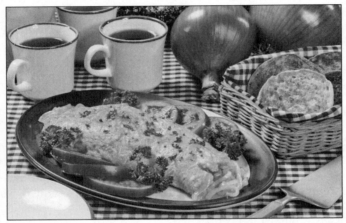

Figure 15-1:
A healthy,
protein-rich
breakfast
starts the
day off right.

Source: PhotoDisc, Inc./Getty Images

If you are a vegetarian, tell your doctors so you can talk about getting appropriate levels of protein from your diet. Also, if your religion prohibits the eating of certain foods, check with your doctors about what substitutes have the highest protein levels.

When your immune system is compromised for extended periods during treatments, you want to avoid eating raw meat, raw fish, and raw eggs. The bacteria in raw foods may cause trouble for you, even if you have suffered no ill effects in the past.

Embracing carbohydrates and fats

This is no time to take up a diet that restricts carbohydrates — in fact, this is not the time to follow any weight-loss plan. We're not saying that you should head for the bakery and pig out, but restrictive eating plans do not serve you well when undergoing treatments for cancer. The body needs carbohydrates to function properly, especially now. Look for carbohydrates in foods such as the following:

- ✔ Fruits
- ✔ Vegetables
- ✔ Bread
- ✔ Pasta
- ✔ Grains
- ✔ Cereals

The body also needs fats to allow the digestive system to work properly. Most people don't need directions to good sources of fats, but here you are:

- ✔ Butter
- ✔ Margarine
- ✔ Oils
- ✔ Nuts
- ✔ Seeds

Whether you prefer butter, margarine, or olive oil, you may continue to use your favorite during your treatments. And remember that meat, fish, and poultry also are sources of fat. For that matter, so is chocolate. The fat in chocolate comes primarily from *stearic acid,* which has a neutral effect on cholesterol. You may have read that chocolate, especially dark chocolate, is good for you in small amounts. Dark chocolate contains *flavonoids,* which researchers say may reduce the harmful effects of LDL — "bad" cholesterol — and may lower blood pressure. Hey, this is science!

Some lab studies suggest that cocoa flavonoids may also reduce the growth of cancer cells. Okay, if you are reading this book, it's too late to take that into consideration, but the point here is that if you enjoy chocolate, indulge yourself from time to time during treatments. In addition to the fat and flavonoids, chocolate contains a chemical known as *tryptophan.* The brain uses tryptophan to make serotonin, which in turn produces feelings of joy and well-being — just what the doctor ordered!

Mulling over vitamins and minerals

Ideally, a well-balanced diet that features fresh, seasonal foods provides plenty of vitamins and minerals that help the body make good use of the calories coming in. In fact, the American Dietetic Association holds that if your diet is what it should be, there is no need for expensive vitamin and mineral supplements. Still, eating a healthy, balanced diet may not be possible as you go through radiation therapy or chemotherapy — or both. Talk with your doctors about whether vitamin and mineral supplements may help you in your effort to get the best nutrition.

Plumbing the Pitfalls of Poor Eating

What happens if you don't eat well? One result may be malnutrition, which means that your body lacks key nutrients. When you are malnourished, you feel weak and tired. Infections have a field day, taking hold and refusing to let go. And when you are malnourished, your treatments are that much harder to endure.

Malnutrition often is a result of one of two conditions. *Anorexia,* or loss of appetite, is the most common. The second is *cachexia,* or wasting syndrome, which leads to loss of weight, fat, and muscle. Sometimes, the two conditions work as a pair, wearing down the body and creating real health problems. Furthermore, cachexia is difficult to reverse.

Not everybody loses weight when going through cancer treatments. In fact, some people gain weight. It depends on what kind of cancer you have, the particular treatment you receive, how well you manage your side effects, and how vigilant you are about eating well.

But we don't want to imply that everyone has complete control over their nutritional health during cancer treatments. Just having cancer causes changes to your body, and treatments for different kinds of cancer also can weaken your will to eat. We discuss these issues next.

Considering Problems that May Develop

A host of nutritional problems can develop from changes caused by having a tumor, having surgery, and having treatments. In this section, we explore some of the most common.

Realizing how tumors impact nutrients

Some tumors produce chemicals that change how the body uses certain nutrients. Tumors of the stomach or intestines, particularly, may affect your body's use of protein, carbohydrates, and fat. Even though you may eat healthy meals, the presence of the tumor may prevent your body from absorbing the nutrients. If that is the case, your doctors likely will recommend more protein and more calories to help prevent the onset of cachexia, or wasting.

Seeing how surgery affects eating habits

More than half of all people diagnosed with cancer go through surgery. Some people, including those with cancers of the head, neck, stomach, and intestines, may go into surgery malnourished. And everyone who goes under the knife needs extra nutrients afterward, because good nutrition helps the body fight infection and recover more quickly.

The problem is that many people experience eating or digestive problems after surgery. Some of the problems are temporary, but some surgeries carry specific challenges. The National Cancer Institute reports the following:

✔ Problems chewing and swallowing may occur after surgery to the head and neck.

✔ Mental stress may affect appetite after surgery, especially if a good deal of tissue has been removed.

✔ The digestive system may not work properly after surgery, especially if organs in the digestive system were removed. For instance, removal of part of the stomach may cause a false feeling of fullness before enough food has been eaten. Also, *dumping syndrome* — emptying of the stomach into the intestines before food is digested — may develop.

✔ If those organs in the digestive system that produce hormones and chemicals necessary for digestion are involved in the surgery, the body may not be able to absorb protein, fat, vitamins, and minerals in the diet, which can lead to imbalances of sugar, salt, and fluid levels.

Cancer-related surgery of any sort may cause fatigue, pain, and loss of appetite. When you begin to get your appetite back, conventional wisdom (along with the National Cancer Institute) recommends the following:

✔ **Avoid carbonated drinks and gas-producing foods.** Think beans, peas, broccoli, cabbage, Brussels sprouts, green peppers, radishes, and cucumbers. Also, if constipation plagues you, drink lots of water and slowly increase the amount of fiber you eat. Fiber is found in oatmeal, bran, beans, vegetables, fruit, and whole-grain breads.

✔ **Eat high protein and high calorie foods.** You have many to choose from, including eggs, cheese, whole milk, ice cream, nuts, peanut butter, meat, poultry, and fish.

✔ **Get out the frying pan.** Frying foods adds fat to the meal, which is recommended at this time. You also may indulge in gravy, mayonnaise, and high fat salad dressings.

Sometimes, either before or after surgery (or both), nutritional supplements are in order. Your doctors will recommend them when such supplements would provide the extra boost you need. Nutritional supplement drinks are available over the counter at most groceries and pharmacies. If that doesn't do it, you may need to be fed liquids through a tube into the stomach or intestine or through a catheter into the bloodstream. Also, appetite-stimulating drugs are available.

Knowing how chemotherapy influences nutrition

Chemotherapy is a systemic treatment that suffuses every nook and cranny of the body. In the drugs' quest to stop or kill completely those cells that divide rapidly, chemotherapy neglects to distinguish between cancer cells and normal, healthy cells. Some of the healthy cells wiped out include cells in the mouth and digestive tract, and that unfortunate circumstance may lead to problems with eating and digestion. See Chapters 10 and 11 for detailed descriptions of possible side effects, including

✔ Nausea and vomiting

✔ Diarrhea or constipation

✔ Inflammation and sores in the mouth

✔ Changes in the way food tastes

✔ Infections

The fatigue that accompanies chemotherapy also may cause you to lose your appetite. Again, nutritional supplements may be in order — either over-the-counter products (usually in liquid form) or liquids fed through a tube into the stomach or intestine, known as *enteral therapy*.

Acknowledging problems caused by radiation therapy

Radiation therapy is site-specific and uses high energy x-rays or other types of radiation to kill cancer cells. Side effects that are directly related to nutrition generally occur when the radiation therapy is aimed at any part of the digestive system. For instance:

- ✔ If your head or neck is involved, you may experience anorexia, changes in taste, dry mouth, inflammation of the mouth and gums, problems swallowing, jaw spasms, cavities, or infection.

- ✔ If your chest is treated, you may get an infection in the esophagus, have problems swallowing, experience *esophageal reflux* (a backwards flow of the stomach contents into the esophagus), nausea, or vomiting.

- ✔ If your abdomen or pelvis is involved, you may have diarrhea, nausea and vomiting, inflammation of the intestine or rectum, or *fistula* (holes) in the stomach or intestines.

- ✔ The fatigue that accompanies most radiation therapy also may cause you to lose your appetite. Again, nutrition therapy may be called for, in the form of over-the-counter supplement drinks, tube feedings, or specific changes in diet. For instance, eating numerous small meals throughout the day may help.

Be sure to discuss each and every symptom with your doctor.

Assessing effects of bone marrow and stem cell transplants

In Chapter 9, we discuss the miracle that is bone marrow and stem cell transplantation. These treatments involve wiping out cells destroyed by cancer treatments with higher doses of chemotherapy or radiation therapy. Then, healthy, cancer-free stem cells are removed from the bone marrow of the patient or a donor, frozen until the time of the transplant, and reintroduced into the body with the hope of restoring the body's supply of blood cells.

If you are scheduled for a bone marrow and stem cell transplant, you are subject to all the nutrition-related side effects that chemotherapy and radiation therapy bring, and you may expect additional side effects from the medications used in the transplant process. These side effects may include

- ✔ Taste changes
- ✔ Dry mouth

✔ Thickened saliva

✔ Mouth and throat sores

✔ Nausea and vomiting

✔ Diarrhea

✔ Constipation

✔ Lack of appetite

✔ Weight gain

Though the list may seem overwhelming, nutrition therapy can successfully treat most of these side effects. The National Cancer Institute notes that nutrition therapy during the transplant process may include the following:

✔ A diet of only cooked and processed foods (no raw vegetables or fresh fruit)

✔ Instruction on safe food handling to avoid infection from food-borne illnesses

✔ Specific diet guidelines based on the type of transplant and the cancer site

✔ *Enteral nutrition* (tube feeding) or *parenteral nutrition* (feeding through the bloodstream) during the first few weeks after the transplant to ensure you get the calories, protein, vitamins, minerals, and fluids needed for good health

Most people being treated for cancer do not experience every possible side effect, especially those that are nutrition-related. As we say elsewhere in this book, every individual responds differently to cancer treatments, so don't count on having to cope with everything that can go wrong. Also, you need not self-prescribe or self-dose to treat nutritional malfunctions. You are not alone in this journey through cancer treatments. You have a team!

Chapter 16

Meeting Spiritual Needs: Turning to Prayer and Meditation

In This Chapter

▶ Confronting spiritual distress

▶ Using spirituality to cope with cancer

▶ Expressing your spirituality to your doctors

▶ Examining different styles of prayer and meditation

▶ Considering one doctor's point of view on spirituality

---

*M*edical treatments help your body fight cancer. Books like this one provide plenty of information for your mind. But what about the needs of your spirit? How do you reconcile cancer with your hopes and dreams, with all that gives rich meaning to your life? These are big questions, and each individual's answers are different, just as each individual approaches spirituality differently.

For some, spirituality is a serene sense of connectedness, achieved by observing order at work in the universe as nature, in the most literal sense, takes its course. For others, spirituality lives within the context of religion and in age-old rituals that hold great meaning for many people around the world. Both sorts of people may turn to prayer or meditation for solace when facing a life-threatening illness, and both are at risk for "spiritual distress," a state of mind that may include guilt, a loss of faith, or a sudden feeling that life has no meaning.

Susan Cuddihee, a hospice chaplain in St. Louis, assures the people with whom she works that "you use your spiritual strength to get through periods of spiritual distress." We all know what our strengths are, but in times of stress — and, certainly, distress — sometimes we forget. Not only do we forget the answers to the big questions, but we forget the questions themselves. Sometimes, we need someone to remind us how we got through challenges in the past and to urge us on by asking how we can use now what we learned then.

In this chapter, we invite you to consider adding a religious and/or spiritual leader to your support team.

Defining Distress

Cancer causes stress. Cancer also causes distress, which can be defined as strong feelings or emotions that may hinder your ability to cope with treatments and with the demands of daily life. Some people feel scared, sad, or powerless — all signs of a mild level of distress. People who are depressed, anxious, or panic-stricken are considered at a high level of distress.

The National Comprehensive Cancer Network reports that surveys done in outpatient clinics show that between 20 and 40 percent of patients have "significant levels of distress." For purposes of evaluating distress, doctors have grouped potential problems into the following categories:

- Physical problems
- Practical problems
- Family problems
- Emotional problems
- Spiritual or religious concerns

If you are experiencing distress, one or more of these problems may be related to past experiences that have colored your ability to cope now. Maybe someone in your family died of cancer. Maybe you have suffered a recent loss of some kind. Maybe you've been treated for depression in the past. Maybe you have even had suicidal thoughts in the past and find those thoughts rushing forward once again.

You want to report problems in any of these areas to your doctors so they can help you. Sometimes, help comes in the form of a referral to a social worker, nutritional expert, or religious or spiritual leader. The last, of course, is particularly qualified to help if you are questioning the faith and religious beliefs that previously provided comfort for you.

Tallying Up the Benefits of Faith

If you are a person of faith, you already know that religion and spirituality provide benefits for your life (see Figure 16-1). Countless polls have reached the same conclusion, noting that people who consider themselves spiritual

"Set free in a dangerous world"

Pat Schneider — an author, poet, and spiritual being living in Amherst, Massachusetts — has a theory about facing difficult times. First, it helps to know that Schneider, 70, says, "My way of finding my way through the multi-layered religious matters is to see everything as holy."

In her book *Wake Up Laughing: A Spiritual Autobiography* (Amherst Writers & Artists Press), Schneider writes:

> *A person's life, like the earth, has its seasons; its griefs and moments of ecstasy are openings into new depths of understanding. . . . We are, each one of us, infinitely loved. Our happiness is longed for. We are each seen and known and called by name. That we are set loose in a wild world where nature, cruelty and accident can injure us does not mean that we are not loved, or that we are of no value.*

> *When my children were infants, an older woman friend advised me to keep them in the playpen until they were four years old. I could not do that. Even though they would have been saved bumps and scratches — perhaps my four-year-old daughter would not have lost the sight in one eye — I had to let them walk away from me in a dangerous world. I tried to keep them company for as long as they would allow me to do so. If I did not set them free, they would not become themselves.*

> *We are set free in a dangerous world. But we are not alone in it. We are each held in a most gracious and loving personal attention. It breathes through this natural world and in our dreams and in our visions. It calls us to respond with love for all living things, to compassion and to work for a world where none of us is alone, none of us is lost.*

or religious report enhanced quality of life. *American Psychologist* — a professional trade publication for those in the field — carried a report in January 2003 by researchers Lynda Powell, Lila Shahabi, and Carl Thoresen saying that "religion and spirituality can provide psychological comfort."

That comfort comes in handy, as it happens, in sickness and in health. According to the American Cancer Society, the U.S. Office of Technology Assessment (OTA) reports that a survey spanning ten years of issues of the *Journal of Family Practice* found that "83 percent of studies on religiosity found a positive effect on physical health." There's more: "Another study on 12 years of issues of two major psychiatric journals found that for the studies that measured religiosity, 92 percent showed a benefit for mental health, 4 percent were neutral, and 4 percent showed harm." According to the American Cancer Society, "religiosity" was measured "by participation in religious ceremony, social support, prayer, and belief in a higher being."

Some data is even more specific. The National Cancer Institute suggests that a positive attitude based on a strong faith or spirituality may provide benefits to people facing cancer, among them:

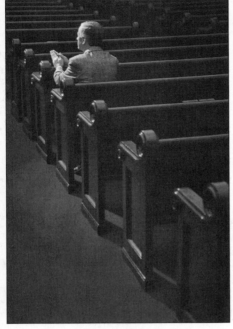

Figure 16-1:
Many
people
report that
spirituality
and religion
improve
their quality
of life.

Source: © Getty Images/Comstock Images

- ✔ Reduced anxiety, depression, and discomfort
- ✔ A decreased sense of feeling alone
- ✔ Better adjustment to the effects of cancer and its treatment
- ✔ An increased ability to enjoy life during cancer treatment
- ✔ A feeling of personal growth as a result of living with cancer
- ✔ Improved health outcomes

Conversely, spiritual distress, or a crisis of faith as a result of being diagnosed, may contribute to a more negative reaction to disease. If your doctor senses such a crisis, she may suggest that you seek guidance from spiritual or religious leaders.

On the other hand, why wait for your doctor to "sense" spiritual distress?

The more information your doctors have about any problems or concerns on your part, the better able they are to help. Spiritual matters are no exception, so don't be afraid to speak up.

Talking about Spirituality with Your Doctors

Some doctors initiate the conversation about spiritual matters by asking what role religion or spirituality plays in your life. Knowing the answer to that question may help your doctors understand your needs — and your reactions — as treatment progresses.

Other doctors may be cautious about bringing up the issue of religious beliefs for fear of offending some patients. If your religion is important to you, you may have to raise the topic yourself. Most doctors will respond positively and ask follow-up questions after you let them know that your spirituality is an important component of who you are. Depending on your needs, the conversation may be short, or it may turn into what the National Cancer Institute calls a "spiritual assessment," designed to assist your doctors. Such an assessment likely would begin with the obvious question, "What religious denomination, if any, are you?" and proceed something like this:

✔ What are your beliefs or philosophy of life?

✔ What important spiritual practices or rituals do you embrace?

✔ Do you use spirituality or religion as a source of strength, and if so, how?

✔ What is your level of participation in a religious community?

✔ How do you use prayer or meditation?

✔ Have you experienced a loss of faith as a result of your cancer diagnosis?

✔ Do you anticipate conflicts between your spiritual or religious beliefs and your cancer treatments?

✔ How can your doctors or nurses address your spiritual needs?

✔ Has cancer caused you to have concerns about death and the afterlife?

✔ Has cancer caused you to think about end-of-life planning, should we come to that point?

You may think such an assessment goes too far, or you may think it doesn't go far enough. Both responses are acceptable, and either makes your conversation with your doctors more meaningful. In other words, feel free to cut the conversation short or to bring up other related questions that have not been addressed. This is one topic where your doctors will look to you to take the lead.

Just as you expect your medical caregivers to respect your views on religion and spirituality, they hope you will return the courtesy by not attempting to debate religious beliefs.

With your spiritual needs and religious views in mind, your doctors are better equipped to make medical decisions consistent with your views and also to support your methods of spiritual coping during treatment. That said, as individuals, your doctors may or may not feel comfortable helping you cope spiritually. As a doctor we know once said, "We have learned to treat people who are ill and we are learning to cry with them, but we have not begun to learn how to pray with them."

Examining Prayer Practices

Prayer takes many forms. Some standard prayers are said at specific times of day or on certain days of the week. Some prayers are spoken aloud, in unison with others in a church, temple, or mosque. Some prayers are whispered when alone. Some are set sequences of words, and others take the form of casual conversation.

Personalizing prayers

Author Anne Lamott favors casual conversation. In her book *Traveling Mercies: Some Thoughts on Faith* (Pantheon), Lamott writes, "Here are the two best prayers I know: 'Help me, help me, help me' and 'Thank you, thank you, thank you.'" Lamott also writes about a friend whose morning prayer is "Whatever" and whose evening prayer is "Oh, well." The late French philosopher and poet Simone Weil wrote, "Absolute attention is prayer," and certainly, "absolute attention" is what you get when you've been diagnosed with cancer.

Praying in free verse

Some songs are prayers, as are some poems. Author Pat Schneider sees the world through new eyes — green-colored glasses, in a sense — in this poem from her book *Another River: New and Selected Poems* (Amherst Writers & Artists Press):

Afternoon of the Day When Doctors First Say 'Cancer'

Oh, green —

Oh green, green, green

Basil and oak and sycamore, more,

More green, and green, and green

Oh pine trees and Oh ghosts of chestnuts,

Oh hickory, sassafras, spinach

And kale green Oh green first

Blade of onion. Oh corn, Oh cucumber,

Lettuce, green lawn,

Oh grass, green moss, Oh green,

Green.

Schneider says the poem is an intense celebration of the present moment. It also reads like a prayer requesting that the author be permitted to stick around long enough to rejoice not only in the greens of the world, but all the other colors as well.

Meditating in a prayerful manner

In some ways, Schneider's poem is a meditation on green. In Chapter 14, we talk about meditation as a worthy way of reducing stress while undergoing treatments. Meditation also can serve as prayer, to soothe the spirit and invite healing. The Cancer Resource Center at the University of California at San Francisco offers weekly drop-in meditation and guided imagery sessions for people going through treatments. The Center recommends meditation for "a variety of beneficial purposes," including gaining self-awareness and personal insight, two benefits that may help ease spiritual distress.

Some meditations begin and end with an intention, such as healing. With this method, you simply quiet yourself and sit still in your own home, gently willing your mind to embrace good health. Guided meditations — led by a class leader or available on a CD or tape — encourage you to visualize yourself as healthy and free of cancer. Some depict the death and disposal of dying cancer cells, but others emphasize instead a vision of warm, healing light.

Some people insist they cannot visualize anything, claiming they don't have a talent for it. But who among us has not anticipated different scenarios that may or may not occur at business meetings, in class, or in social situations? That, my friend, is a type of visualization. If you can do that, you may benefit from guided meditation.

Some meditation CDs and tapes consist of instrumental music with sounds of nature — no voices — woven in among the notes. If you try one that doesn't suit you, we encourage you to try another.

Accepting Prayers from Others

Whatever form they take — conversations, attention, songs, poems, or meditation — some prayers are for the self, and some, known as *intercessory prayers,* are for others. Some of these prayers "for others" may come your way as you undergo treatments. Many churches and synagogues have prayer lists that they read aloud each week at services, or sometimes, members of the congregation rise and speak the names of people in need of prayers. Count yourself lucky if you get on these lists.

Many people of many different faiths freely offer prayers for friends going through cancer treatments. Regardless of your religious or spiritual beliefs, we believe the best response is a heartfelt "thank you" in acknowledgement of a thoughtful gift.

These gifts do come from the heart. As noted in an article on prayer and science by Benedict Carey published October 10, 2004, in *The New York Times,* "Some researchers point out that praying for the relief of other people's suffering is a deeply human response to disease."

Assessing the Healing Power of Prayer

Can prayer heal illness?

Since 2004, the federal government has spent $2.3 million to finance prayer research under the auspices of the National Center for Complementary and Alternative Medicine, which is part of the National Institutes of Health. That expense, and the topic in general, are both controversial. "For one thing," Benedict Carey writes in *The New York Times,* "No one knows what constitutes a 'dose': some studies have tested a few prayers a day by individual healers, while others have had entire congregations pray together. Some have involved evangelical Christians; others have engaged rabbis, Buddhist and New Age healers, or some combination."

To date, studies have engaged individuals to pray for people with heart disease, AIDS, brain tumors, fertility problems, and a number of other diseases and conditions. The American Cancer Society notes that "although research has not shown that spirituality can cure cancer or any other disease, some studies have found intercessory prayer may be an effective addition to conventional medical care." The organization cites a study conducted in San Francisco in 1988 that showed that "seriously ill patients who were prayed for were less likely to need antibiotics and had fewer complications." A second study conducted in Kansas City reported similar findings.

Though the results of the studies suggest that "prayer may be an effective complementary therapy to conventional medical treatment," the American Cancer Society also issues this cautionary note: Choosing to avoid conventional medical care in favor of prayer alone may result in serious health consequences.

Listening to a Doctor on Spirituality

Still, we're not about to come out against the value of prayer or meditation, whether personal or intercessory. Science and religion often work as partners. For instance, many medical centers have chaplains on staff, chapels in the building, and business arrangements with ministers, rabbis, and other religious and spiritual leaders to serve patients. At least one high-profile doctor has made it his business to research the relationship between prayer and healing.

Dr. Larry Dossey, originally a specialist in internal medicine from Texas, also served for a time as chief of staff at Medical City Dallas Hospital and was co-chair of the panel on Mind/Body Interventions in the Office of Alternative Medicine at the National Institutes of Health. He most recently served as executive editor of the publication *Alternative Therapies in Health and Medicine*.

Dr. Dossey is the author of nine books, among them *Healing Beyond the Body* (Shambhala), *Reinventing Medicine* (Harper), *Prayer is Good Medicine* (Harper), and *Healing Words* (Harper). He also has written numerous articles on this topic and lectures around the world. We include him in this chapter not as an endorsement, but simply to present his interesting point of view.

Considering the historical perspective

Dr. Dossey is not the first "medicine man" to discuss the spiritual art of healing and the science of medicine in the same sentence. For thousands of years, many cultures relied on individuals who served as spiritual leaders and physicians at the same time. These individuals, honored and held in high regard, were known as priest-healers, shamans, and faith healers. Sometimes, these individuals came directly to the ill; other times, sick people were brought to temples for healing. The healers of the day used herbs and other plant extracts combined with mind-altering drugs and intoxicants, all mixed together with a hearty dose of the power of suggestion.

Sometimes, it worked — and in some ways, that's still the case today, as medical science continues to advance.

According to Dr. Dossey, "[W]hen used in tandem with other orthodox and alternative measures, prayer is indeed powerful medicine." On his Web site at www.dosseydossey.com, Dr. Dossey also is quoted saying that "[P]rayer is remarkably democratic: Research confirms that no particular religion holds a monopoly on prayer's efficacy; and one does not need to be religious, per se, to pray effectively or to benefit medically from prayer."

Now, that's spiritual news you can use.

Squaring Faith with Cancer

Maybe you think of yourself as both spiritual and religious, or maybe you use just one of these terms to describe yourself. Maybe you use neither. In any case, cancer likely has rocked your world. Some people become angry when diagnosed with cancer. Some feel they are being punished. Some appear to take the diagnosis in stride, saying cancer is a burden they can bear. And sometimes, one individual experiences all three states of mind, by turns.

Do you ask, "Why me?" Or do you figure, "Why not me?" Which is the correct question, the right attitude? The answers are not in this chapter or elsewhere in this book. The best we can do is remind you that in scientific terms, cancer is a disease that most often responds to medical treatment. However, we hope that the material we've provided in this chapter is thought-provoking regarding the role of spirituality in coping with cancer.

Chapter 17

Finding a Support Group: Realizing You Are Not Alone

*A*t this point, your support team is so big — family, friends, doctors, nurses, additional health professionals, and spiritual or religious leaders — that you would need a bus should you decide to transport them all to one place at one time. Better call for a second bus. Some of the most meaningful help available when you have cancer may come from a group of complete strangers.

What can a cancer support group do for you that no one else can do? The members can silently nod as you speak of your experience, and then they can look you in the eye and say, "I know how you feel. I've been there."

That nod, that direct gaze, that affirmation of your emotions simply is not available anywhere else. You say you aren't interested in talking about your cancer with a bunch of strangers? That's okay, because today, some support groups meet online. You miss the eye contact, of course, but the empathy and the sense that "we're all in this together" come through.

In this chapter, we consider the benefits and risks of support groups and help you figure out whether you are interested in adding another dozen or so exceptionally qualified people to your support team.

Determining Your Level of Interest

Maybe you've had experience with other support groups, so you know what to expect. Or maybe you have never been in a situation that required even thinking about being part of a support group. If that's the case, here are some questions that may help you sort out whether you would find a support group appealing:

- ✔ Are you comfortable being part of a group?
- ✔ Do you enjoy the give and take of a group?
- ✔ Are you comfortable talking about your feelings in front of people outside your immediate circle?
- ✔ Are you willing to listen to the experiences and concerns of other people going through treatments?
- ✔ Are you inclined to listen to advice from people who already have been through cancer treatments?
- ✔ Do you think you may be able to provide advice to others?
- ✔ Are you comfortable in the company of other people who have had cancer?
- ✔ Are you able to calmly agree to disagree?
- ✔ Do you view your doctors as the only reliable sources of information about cancer and treatments?

This isn't a quiz, though it may sound like it. There are no right or wrong answers, but these questions may help you determine how well you would function in a cancer support group.

Support groups are not for everyone. If you have a strong support network among family and friends and have no interest in allowing thoughts of cancer to take up one more minute of your time, feel free to skip to the next chapter.

Defining "Group"

In this case, "group" has multiple meanings. How many people are in a typical support group? That depends on the group you choose. Some groups present monthly programs, where you may find yourself seated in a room with three dozen other people all on hand to hear a featured speaker talk about some aspect of cancer. Weekly groups led by licensed therapists or trained peer counselors generally have ten or fewer members (see Figure 17-1).

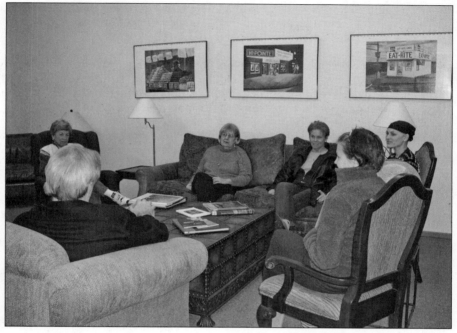

Figure 17-1:
Support from other people going through cancer treatments can be valuable.

Source: The Wellness Community of Greater St. Louis

And some support programs pair you with just one other person, someone who has experienced the same kind of cancer that you have. In this case, you represent half of a group of two, with the option of talking on the phone as often or as little as needed. Online, of course, you have no idea how many people may be reading or considering responding to what you have to say.

Who comes to a support group? You may think the answer to that question is as obvious as the answer to the question about who is buried in Grant's tomb, but it's not. Some groups are restricted to people going through cancer. Others welcome spouses, family members, or other members of a support team.

With so many "groups" to choose from, you're likely to find one that appeals to you and meets your needs.

Locating a Group

These days, it's almost impossible not to trip over any number of support groups. Some are open only to people with one kind of cancer, and others bring together people diagnosed with all different kinds. Psychologists and/or social workers lead some groups, and peer counselors lead others. Some groups meet only online. The advantage there is that a listening ear is available 24 hours a day, seven days a week.

If you look for support online, consider using a pseudonym or just your initials to identify yourself. Also, be wary of any advice regarding medications or herbal remedies. The person recommending the same may work for a drug company or be a salesperson promoting a product.

Think about what sort of group may best meet your needs, and ask your doctors or nurses or talk with a social worker or cancer education specialist at your hospital for some recommendations. We bet you will get what you need from them, but if you don't, here are some places to look for resources:

- ✔ Large medical centers
- ✔ Local branches of national cancer organizations or service agencies (such as the American Cancer Society or The Wellness Community)
- ✔ Churches or places of worship
- ✔ Web sites devoted to specific kinds of cancer

Saluting The Wellness Community

The Wellness Community is a national nonprofit organization operating in almost two dozen cities (with five more centers in development) and also in Israel and Japan. The organization "provides support, education and hope" to people of all ages with cancer and to their loved ones in a homelike setting that features plenty of comfortable couches and chairs, as well as boxes of tissues on every table. The Wellness Community offers support groups, as well as classes in a variety of subjects including yoga, relaxation, spirituality, nutrition, and the expressive arts. The organization also features special programs and, occasionally, holds parties. All the programs are free.

Dr. Harold Benjamin of Santa Monica founded The Wellness Community in 1982 after helping his wife go through breast cancer and then studying the psychological and social impact of cancer. Today, people who show up at The Wellness Community's doors include people newly diagnosed, people undergoing treatment, people experiencing recurrence, and people several years past treatment. In 2003, The Wellness Community reached more than 30,000 people affected by cancer, who attended more than 200,000 support group sessions and programs.

This successful organization, which serves as a model for programs throughout the United States, also conducts research "to quantify and document the benefits of psychosocial support for people with cancer." Partners in this research include Catholic University, M.D. Anderson Cancer Center, Rutgers University, Stanford University, the University of California at Los Angeles, and the University of California at San Francisco.

As we write this, The Wellness Community is operating in Atlanta, Ga.; Boca Raton, Fla.; Boston, Mass.; Cincinnati, Ohio; Columbus, Ohio; Indianapolis, Ind.; Knoxville, Tenn.; Miami, Fla.; Orange County, Calif.; Pasadena, Calif.; Philadelphia, Pa.; Phoenix, Ariz.; Redondo Beach, Calif.; Salisbury, Md.; San Francisco, Calif.; Santa Monica, Calif.; Sarasota, Fla.; St. Louis, Mo.; Valley/Ventura, Calif.; and Wilmington, Del. Additional "satellite" groups meet in hospitals, cancer centers, and community centers near the cities listed here.

You say your city isn't listed here? In 2002, the organization launched "The Virtual Wellness Community," which provides free, professionally led support groups online. For more information on any of The Wellness Community's programs, call 888-793-9355 or 202-659-9709, or visit www.thewellnesscommunity.org.

Support groups vary widely. If you try one and find it doesn't suit you, consider visiting a different group sponsored by a different organization or agency.

First impressions are important, but not always reliable. Sometimes it takes two or three visits to get a good sense of what one particular group is about and to determine whether it answers your needs. Your coauthor Patricia left one group after two visits because "the people there were too quiet, the room was too dark, and the cookies were terrible." She did a bit more "shopping" and found a group at the local branch of The Wellness Community that suited her perfectly. (See the sidebar "Saluting The Wellness Community.")

Asking the Right Questions

After you have found a group that interests you, you may want to quiz the contact person before you attend a meeting. Here are some questions to ask:

- ✔ When and where are the meetings?
- ✔ How long is each meeting?
- ✔ How large is the group?
- ✔ Who comes to the meetings?
- ✔ What is the age range?
- ✔ How many meetings does the average person typically attend?
- ✔ Who leads the meetings?

> ✔ Are the meetings structured around a theme, or do participants bring up topics they want to discuss?
>
> ✔ Is the emphasis on emotional well-being or practical ways to get through treatments?
>
> ✔ Is there a fee to attend?

With answers to these questions in hand, you aren't likely to encounter any surprises at the first meeting you attend. You may even want to ask if you may sit in on a meeting to see how you like it.

Seeking One-on-One Support

If the idea of going through cancer treatments with a group of strangers — whether in person or online — does not appeal to you, a number of organizations will work to put you in touch with an individual close to your age and with a similar background who also was diagnosed with the same kind of cancer. Typically, these individuals are at least one year past diagnosis, and they've participated in a training program for peer counseling.

The sources for such programs are the same as those listed earlier in this chapter in the section "Locating a Group."

Looking at the Benefits

When you have located a support group that appeals to you, you may wonder what's in it for you. That's a fair question! At one time, research indicated that women with breast cancer who attended support groups lived about 18 months longer than those who did not. The results of this study were published in 1989, and probably more than one woman undergoing treatment for breast cancer who had no interest in being part of a support group signed up for meetings anyway.

A study published in *The New England Journal of Medicine* in December 2001 reported quite different results. The Canadian researchers who conducted the study between 1993 and 1998 found that "patients survived about the same length of time whether they took part in a support group or not."

However, Dr. Pamela Goodwin of Mount Sinai Hospital at the University of Toronto did not focus the study strictly on survival. She and her colleagues also asked about the participants' moods and their perceptions of pain.

Goodwin found that the women in group therapy "reported less worsening of pain and had significantly lower scores on measures of depression, anxiety and bewilderment." She also discovered that "women who were highly distressed when they entered the study benefited from group therapy more than women who were initially less distressed."

The essence of Dr. Goodwin's findings is that support groups — at least for women with breast cancer — may enhance quality of life, but women with no interest in taking part in a support group need not feel guilty. That said, the study is part of a body of evidence that shows that support groups offer people with all kinds of cancer the following opportunities:

✔ To be with people who truly understand how you feel

✔ To lighten the burden of having cancer

✔ To talk openly about your feelings about cancer

✔ To cope better with your treatments

✔ To get tips on how to handle fears or unexpected behavior of family members or friends

✔ To give yourself a new perspective on your experience

✔ To increase your confidence about being accepted in spite of physical changes brought on by cancer treatments

Most people who attend support groups acknowledge support from family, friends, and co-workers. What they come looking for and, most often, receive from a group is complete acceptance of any fear, feeling, mood, or attitude in place on the day of the meeting.

Support groups provide an opportunity for you to remove any mask you may feel compelled to wear at home, at work, or in the company of others who have never had cancer. That benefit alone is significant beyond words.

Assessing the Risks

Now you know some of the important benefits of taking part in a support group. The flip side is the risks. The risks are not physical, unless you fear that attending the meetings will increase your level of fatigue. The risks are psychological, and meetings may mess with your emotional equilibrium.

Handling the hard stuff

In addition to the warm acceptance, practical tips, sense of belonging, and much spontaneous laughter that you likely will experience at a support group, you also may witness outright anger or fear. You may hear sad stories about spouses walking out, parents who can't cope, and bosses who choose to make life miserable for people going through cancer treatments. And you may, as the weeks ago by, watch someone approach death.

Can you handle all that?

As much as you want to talk about your fears, you may find that listening to someone else's is hard for you. As much as you want to rejoice with the man who danced at his daughter's wedding, something he thought he never would be able to do, you may not care to hear the sobs of the young woman as she reports that her fiancé has left her. One person in the group may say exactly what you need to hear the very night you need to hear it (in Patricia's case, it was that she needed to stop trying so hard to be the "perfect cancer patient"). But that same night, another person may wonder aloud what you did to "deserve" cancer and throw you into an emotional tailspin.

Protecting yourself emotionally

If you commit to attending a support group, early on you will learn to practice separation exercises, to differentiate in no uncertain terms between your situation and that of others.

When you're sitting in a room next to a person trying to come to grips with a traumatic situation in his life, sometimes it's easy to take on that person's problems, to be drawn into that person's drama, and to carry that person's burdens home with you from the support group.

Not to sound cold, but this is no time to borrow trouble. You have your own life-threatening situation and possible complications at home or at work to handle.

Empathy, certainly, and expressions of concern for the person sitting next to you are in order, if you are indeed moved by his story and wish to offer words of support. That fulfills your obligation.

One of the best ways to keep other people's problems in perspective is to remind yourself silently, "This is me, sitting here. The person going through such a hard time is sitting over there. Though we may have a cancer diagnosis in common, that's not me. I'm sitting here." By concentrating on the physical separation, you can maintain a healthier emotional separation. This is no cop-out, but an important method of protection.

Your role as a member of a support group is not to fix another person's problems. You fulfill every obligation, if there is one, simply by listening sensitively and giving others the opportunity to vent their concerns, fears, and personal trials.

After you have mastered the separation exercise, recognized the subtle way in which you may be helping, and fine-tuned your attitude so that you can hear the hard stuff and listen with empathy, you still may find yourself depressed after any given meeting. If that's the case, you owe it to yourself to drop out.

That doesn't mean you will be on your own. In fact, you likely already have a handpicked support team in place, with every member standing by to help you in any way.

No matter what resources for support you choose to use, you don't have to go through cancer treatments alone.

Helping Newcomers

If you do decide to attend support group meetings or join an online chat group for people undergoing cancer treatments, the day may come that you find yourself focusing not on what the group can do for you but on how you may be able to help someone else.

Remember experiencing that first rush of complete acceptance from other members of the group? At some point, you may be able to repay an emotional "debt" to the group by providing that same level of acceptance, that same sense of relief, for a newcomer. What an emotionally satisfying day that is! When that day comes, you will not necessarily be at a point where you are no longer receiving help and benefiting from your participation. That's a different day, and you will recognize it went it comes.

Some people feel ready to stop participating in a support group more quickly than others, so there is no right or wrong time to expect yourself to leave the group.

You may find significant emotional satisfaction in helping newcomers as they face the same struggles that you so recently have triumphed over. Sticking around to be of help is laudatory, as long as you do it because you want to and not because you think you must. Even after you do leave, you likely will continue to draw on the strength and emotional support that you gained from the group.

Here's another benefit: You may have made some new friends whom you will continue to enjoy meeting with on a social basis. Hey, the rest of your support team gladly will make room for one or two more members.

Part VI
Your Future after Cancer Treatments: Looking Ahead

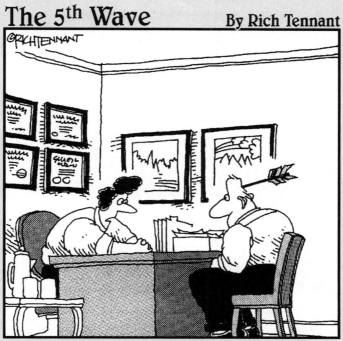

The 5th Wave   By Rich Tennant

"I'm pretty certain what we're dealing with here is not a recurrence of cancer."

In this part . . .

Unexpected roadblocks — such as physical changes, recurrence (or fear of same), and emotional upsets — sometimes pop up after cancer treatments have ended. This part provides a sensible map to help you navigate any speed bumps that may be in your future.

Chapter 18

Finishing Therapy: An End and a Beginning

*H*as it ever occurred to you while sitting through a commencement ceremony that *commencement* isn't exactly the right word to describe the full character of the event? Yes, the students are moving on to a new level of schooling or out into the world, and so they are *commencing* the next stage of life. However, the students also are leaving something behind, and the event itself combines an ending with a beginning.

Finishing cancer treatments also is an occasion that represents an ending but makes way for new beginnings. Just as those students on commencement day look forward to an exciting future but also feel anxious about leaving the known for the unknown, your emotions may be mixed about finishing treatment. That's to be expected. And, just like the students, you won't be making the transition alone.

By now you have probably guessed that on the last day of chemotherapy or radiation, your doctors will not simply shake your hand, say goodbye, and turn you out to fend for yourself. No, you will be carefully monitored for years to come.

In this chapter, you get an idea of what to expect after your treatments end. In Chapter 20, we address emotional issues you may deal with after treatments end. Here, we keep the focus on your physical health.

Monitoring Your Health after Cancer

So you've said goodbye to the medical technicians and the patients with whom you've made friends during radiation therapy, or you've sat for the last time waiting for the last drop of chemotherapy drugs to enter your bloodstream. Now what? Do you just go home and try to forget that you ever had cancer? Not exactly.

You may feel relieved that treatments are over and you're ready to move on. Or you may feel like a soldier left on the battlefield with no weapon to continue fighting your cancer. Bouts of "survivor anxiety" may come and go in the first few months after treatments end. That's normal, and they do lessen over time. (If you think your feelings of anxiety are increasing, by all means make an appointment to speak with your doctor.)

When treatments end, your family and friends may express relief and then expect you to be your old self. You may even expect this yourself. Frankly, that's unrealistic. Cancer and its treatments change your body, and those changes don't disappear overnight. In this section, we show you what to expect during the first weeks, months, and years after your treatments end.

Expecting a recovery period

Before we begin any detailed discussions about follow-up care, long-term side effects, drugs your doctor may prescribe, or anything else, you need to know that most people don't "get over" cancer treatments quickly. Your particular timetable will depend on these factors:

- Your age
- Your general health
- The type of cancer you had
- The treatments you received
- The length of time you were treated
- Your body's reaction to the treatments

It can take a year or more for your body to recover. This doesn't mean that you will feel exactly the same 12 months after treatments end as you felt at your first follow-up appointment. Recovery is a process, and as each month passes, you likely will feel better and enjoy ever-increasing levels of energy and strength.

If your mind is in a rush and encourages you to get back to normal activity levels more quickly than is possible for your body, don't be surprised if your body complains by slowing you down even more.

You are in a recuperation stage. Recovery from cancer treatments takes time. Also, you are older than you were when you first were diagnosed, so your body may have been different at this point even if you had *not* had cancer. Be patient as you work toward the goal of renewed health.

Scheduling follow-up care

Most likely, your medical oncologist and radiation oncologist will provide a schedule of follow-up care for you. The schedule for these follow-up appointments will depend on the kind of cancer you had and what treatments you received, but generally a doctor on your support team may want to see you every three to four months for at least two or three years and then just once or twice a year after that.

Some insurance policies pay for only a certain number of follow-up visits. Check on what your policy allows, and if it is far less often than what your doctor has in mind, ask your doctor to speak with someone at your insurance company.

Chances are you haven't spent much time in your internist's office during cancer treatments, and this may be a good time to set up an appointment. When you see this doctor, you can report on your progress during cancer treatments just in case she has not received recent updates from your medical and radiation oncologists.

If you live a good distance from the oncologist's office, you may prefer to have your follow-up visits with your internist. If that's the case, be sure to talk with both doctors so they know what arrangements you wish to make.

Keeping appointments

No one can blame you at this point if you've had enough of doctors and tests and trips to the medical center for treatments. You probably need a rest, and you certainly deserve one. However, this is no time to make yourself scarce. Monitoring your health after cancer treatments end is serious business, and your doctor can't do a good job if you don't cooperate.

You've already given many months of your life over to cancer treatments. What's a few more? Plan to see this experience through.

The day will come when you will turn the next few pages of your calendar and not see any doctor's appointments, tests, or scans on your schedule, and we have no doubt that you'll have plenty of ideas on how to spend your free time. (See Chapter 20 for some suggestions.) Until then, plan to keep your follow-up appointments and get any tests or scans recommended by your doctor. You're doing yourself a favor. You already know the poignant truth of that old adage, "If you don't have your health, you don't have anything," so make a commitment to stay as healthy as possible.

You may want to take a notebook or tape recorder to your appointments. That way, you'll have a record of any suggestions the doctor makes for you as you navigate the healing process.

Telling the truth

So what happens at a follow-up appointment? First, the doctor asks you how you feel. Be truthful. If you're still tired, have no appetite, or think that your body is not healing, say so. You also want to talk to your doctor about any pain you're feeling.

What else should you talk about? Of course, that depends on what you're experiencing. Prepare for your appointment by considering what questions you want to ask. Here are a few examples to get you thinking:

- ✔ If you've lost your hair, how long will it take for it to grow back?
- ✔ If you received radiation, will the affected skin lighten again?
- ✔ If you're having trouble sleeping, why, and what can you do about it?
- ✔ If your appetite is erratic (one day you're hungry, and the next day you're not), why, and what can you do about it?

Perhaps your arthritis is acting up. Maybe you've noticed a rash on your skin. Or your spouse or partner may have urged you to ask the doctor about a lagging sex drive. Your vision may be cloudy, or maybe your mouth is unusually dry. Whatever is bothering you, be sure to speak up.

During your follow-up visits, mention any changes or troubles you are experiencing concerning your physical or mental health. Cancer treatments affect the entire body, so any symptom or discomfort is fair game when you talk with the oncologist.

Worrying about recurrence

If you are worried that the cancer may come back — and that is a common fear among people who have been treated for cancer — tell the doctor. One woman we know describes this fear as "a dark cloud that follows me around." That cloud often gets bigger and becomes more menacing a day or two before each follow-up appointment, even a year or more after treatments end. However, the cloud also may show up every time you get a cold or a sore throat or a pulled muscle in your leg. If you are the sort who worries in such detail — and this is far more common than you may think — please allow your doctor to hear you out and do what he can to set your mind at ease.

Cancer changes everything, and memories of the experience may well cause you and other survivors to make mountains of what others clearly see as molehills.

Here's the good news: The fear of recurrence fades a little more every time you have a successful follow-up visit and every time you "pass" any test designed to monitor your health. Still, let the doctor know if you are worrying about recurrence. (See Chapter 19 for more information about recurrence.) The two of you then can discuss any symptoms that you need to watch for in between visits or any screening tests that you may need to have. If your level of concern is particularly high, the doctor may order scans or other tests to evaluate the situation.

Coping with Long-Term Side Effects

So here you are, finished with treatments, and yet you're still plagued by side effects. What's the deal? In one sense, the side effects represent lingering protection for you, because their presence means that the treatments are still working in your body. In most cases, the side effects eventually come to an end.

In this section, we discuss some of the common side effects that may linger after treatment ends.

Fighting fatigue

At this point, you're probably tired of being tired. You already know that a good night's sleep failed to lessen the fatigue that you experienced during treatments. When the same holds true after treatments end, you're likely to become frustrated or even angry. Recovering from this level of fatigue takes time. In Chapters 10 and 13, you can find suggestions to help relieve your fatigue. Maybe you already read these suggestions when you were starting chemotherapy or radiation therapy, but this may be a good time to review them.

Putting up with pain

Pain, which can increase feelings of fatigue, may be an unwelcome visitor after treatments end. If you had cancer surgery, the scar may still be uncomfortable, and nearby skin may tingle or "buzz" incessantly. If you had a breast or limb removed, you may feel pain where the body part once was. This sensation is not uncommon, and your doctor likely will regard it as legitimate pain. Sometimes surgery or chemotherapy can lead to pain or numbness in your hands or feet. Also, radiated skin may be exceptionally sensitive.

Seeking relief from these and other types of pain will help you get on the road to recovery sooner, so speak up about any pain that you are experiencing. You may need to take pain medication for a while, or you may need physical therapy. The doctor may suggest that you try meditation or yoga to learn relaxation skills. (See Chapter 14 for more on meditation and yoga.)

Also, don't overlook the power of humor. Laughing at your children's antics or watching a funny movie may provide some temporary relief from pain. That's not wishful thinking — it's science: Laughing causes your brain to release chemicals that lead to muscle relaxation, which may reduce pain.

Managing lymphedema

Lymphedema — a build-up of lymphatic fluid in an arm or a leg — can result from cancer surgery or radiation therapy. (See Chapter 13 for details about lymphedema.) Basically, the earlier that lymphedema is diagnosed and treated, the better the outcome. However, some swelling may stay with you for years to come. Several treatments are available for treating lymphedema, so if swelling is a problem, mention it to your doctor.

Making the best of mouth problems

Almost everyone who has radiation therapy to the head and neck continues to have problems with the mouth or teeth after treatment, and the same can be said for almost half the people who have chemotherapy. Your mouth may be dry or painful, your taste buds may be on strike, or you may find yourself spending a lot of time at the dentist dealing with cavities or other dental problems.

Perhaps you are having trouble swallowing, or you have run out of ideas for finding protein-rich foods that don't irritate your throat. (Again, see Chapters 10 and 13 for helpful suggestions.) You may want to consider investing in commercial powdered protein supplements (which may be mixed with either milk or yogurt) or upping your intake of soft, moist, protein-rich foods such as eggs or dairy products.

This is the time to maximize every calorie that does pass your lips — use butter instead of margarine, put cream in your breakfast cereal instead of milk, and always have a bedtime snack. (In general, forget every rule you may have followed if you've ever tried to watch your weight!)

Report any mouth or throat problems during a follow-up appointment so your doctor knows which long-term side effects are making you uncomfortable. Relief is available, and your doctor may also discuss some preventative measures that may help stop the problem from becoming worse.

Facing bladder or bowel problems

If you were treated for cancer of the bladder, prostate, colon, rectum, or ovaries, you may not have bowel or bladder control, or that control may be limited. This problem can be embarrassing, particularly if you lead an active life. Be upfront about your concerns, and be sure to let your doctor know exactly what challenges you face. Help is available — even if you are dealing with an *ostomy,* which is a surgically constructed excretory opening. Resolving other problems may call for medications, exercise, or even surgery.

Accepting early menopause

Many women who go through chemotherapy — even young women — find themselves thrown into early menopause. No matter what your opinion of menopause is — whether you see it as a normal, healthy part of life or as a disturbing loss of fertility — facing early menopause as a result of cancer treatments can be unsettling. Aside from a woman's emotional response, the physical symptoms of menopause can be challenging. Here are some of the typical symptoms of menopause:

- Irregular periods
- Hot flashes
- Dry, thin vaginal tissues
- Declining sex drive
- Sleep deprivation
- Short-term memory loss
- Mood swings
- Increase in body fat
- Declining elasticity of the skin

Some women, especially younger women, do eventually get their periods again, but many do not. If yours is gone for good and you're having trouble coping with menopause, mention it to your oncologist and also consider making an appointment with your gynecologist, who will have specific suggestions on how to cope with symptoms.

If you had an estrogen-fed cancer — and your doctor can tell you if that is the case — check with your oncologist before filling any prescription for hormone replacement therapy recommended by another physician who may be unaware of your medical history. Hormone replacement therapy, prescribed to ease the symptoms of menopause, may put you at risk for recurrence.

Also, be aware that herbal remedies and soy products that contain *phytoestrogens* — natural plant compounds that act like estrogen in the body — also could lead to increased hormonal activity that could put you at risk for recurrence. The ingestion of phytoestrogens may or may not be an important issue for your type of cancer, so it's worth checking with your doctors before putting soy products and herbal remedies in the shopping bag.

By the way, menopause is not only for females; there is a male equivalent. Some of the cautions and advice we offer in this section may apply to men as well. Ask your doctor about whether your health may potentially be affected before you try any remedy for the symptoms of menopause.

Sorting out sexual issues

During cancer treatments, you probably did not feel particularly sexy or have a lot of interest in a high level of intimacy. Unfortunately, the same may hold true after treatments end.

Research shows that almost half the women treated for breast cancer or cancer of the reproductive organs and more than half the men treated for prostate cancer report long-term problems with intimacy. Sometimes having sex is painful, and sometimes — in the case of some men who have had prostate cancer, cancer of the penis, or cancer of the testes — having sex is simply not possible.

The four main concerns that cancer survivors most often report are

✔ A declining interest in sex

✔ An inability to have sex as before

✔ Menopausal symptoms

✔ Infertility

Time and/or medication may help with the first three issues, but infertility likely will require different approaches. Be bold, and discuss any problems with intimacy and sexuality with your doctor so he can help you whenever possible. Also, don't avoid discussing your problems with your spouse or partner. Together, with plenty of patience, you can work through some of the problems or learn to be intimate in new ways that provide satisfaction for you both.

Reducing Your Hormone Level

In addition to the follow-up appointments and screening tests that you can expect to have after finishing cancer treatments, some people start hormone therapy, which is also known as *endocrine therapy*. This is not the same kind of hormone replacement therapy familiar to women of a certain age. Hormone therapy for cancer is used to reduce the level of hormones in your body or to stop the spread of cancer that depends on your hormones to grow.

Hearing arguments for hormone therapy

Some tumors use estrogen and testosterone, in women and men respectively, to survive and grow. These tumors are called *hormone-fed* or *hormone-responsive* tumors. The doctor does not have to guess whether your tumor falls into this category. Instead, a pathologist performs a biopsy on the tumor, and a sample of tissue is analyzed in a laboratory. If the tumor is found to be hormone-responsive, your medical oncologist likely will recommend hormone therapy in order to cut off the tumor's meal ticket, as it were, by decreasing the hormone level in your body or by blocking the tumor's route to the hormones it wants and needs for growth.

Cancers most likely to be hormone-receptive include

- ✔ Breast cancer
- ✔ Prostate cancer
- ✔ Ovarian cancer
- ✔ Uterine cancer

We mention in Chapter 4 that some forms of hormone therapy are used to treat such cancers as lymphoma, leukemia, and multiple myeloma. Sometimes, hormone therapy also is used to shrink tumors before surgery so they are easier to remove. And sometimes doctors recommend hormone therapy after treatments are over to try to keep your cancer from coming back.

Considering different approaches

Hormone therapy is available in several forms, including surgery, radiation, and drugs:

- ✔ Surgery is the most straightforward but also the most drastic method used to reduce your level of hormones. Possible surgeries include
  - • Removal of the testicles (*orchiectomy* or *castration*)
  - • Removal of the ovaries (*oophorectomy)* in premenopausal women
  - • Removal of the adrenal gland (*adrenalectomy)* in post-menopausal women
  - • Removal of the pituitary gland (*hypophysectomy)* in women

  In those instances when a choice is available, most people prefer to take hormone-suppressive drugs rather than have surgery.
- ✔ Radiation therapy can stop hormone production in the testicles, ovaries, and adrenal and pituitary glands.
- ✔ Drug therapy can be used to block the access of cancer cells to your body's supply of estrogen or testosterone. Some drugs may be taken in pill form or as an injection.

Sizing up the side effects

Side effects reported by men and women undergoing hormone therapy differ somewhat. Generally, men report the following side effects:

- ✔ Decrease in sexual desire
- ✔ Enlarged breasts
- ✔ Hot flashes
- ✔ Inability to achieve an erection
- ✔ Incontinence
- ✔ Osteoporosis

Women tend to experience side effects that mimic common symptoms of menopause, including

- ✔ Fatigue
- ✔ Hot flashes
- ✔ Mood swings
- ✔ Nausea
- ✔ Osteoporosis
- ✔ Weight gain

Unfortunately, over time, some cancer cells become resistant to hormone therapy and find a way to grow even without the hormones that the cells originally depended upon. If your cancer cells outsmart your hormone drugs, you still have options. A different drug may rise to the occasion and take over the task of keeping estrogen and progesterone from feeding developing tumors.

Besides hormone therapies, additional maintenance strategies to fend off recurrence also are available for some kinds of cancer. Ask your doctor about drugs for certain types of lymphoma, post-induction therapy for leukemia, and aspirin for survivors of early colorectal cancer.

Deciding what's best for you

As always, we recommend that you talk with your doctor about all your options and about the side effects of each type of hormone therapy. Consider, too, the benefits of the different treatments and which best fits your lifestyle now that you have finished with chemotherapy and radiation treatments.

Working Out a Wellness Plan

When your principal treatments are over, no matter how many side effects linger, you may find yourself intensely interested in how to achieve and maintain good health. You also likely will want to know what to do to avoid recurrence or reduce your risk of getting a different kind of cancer. In Chapter 2, we write in detail about some of the common risk factors for cancer and some of the recommendations to help reduce risk. These recommendations, of course, apply to people who have never been diagnosed with cancer.

Researchers have not yet determined whether specific health practices will prevent recurrence or development of a new cancer after you have already had the disease.

Still, you may want to acquaint yourself with these recommendations, and introduce them — one by one, if you choose, or all at once — into your life. Here, in brief, are some of the health practices that may reduce the risk of certain kinds of cancer:

- ✔ Stop smoking
- ✔ Exercise regularly
- ✔ Drink alcohol in moderation
- ✔ Eat a well-balanced diet
- ✔ Protect your skin from the sun
- ✔ Avoid exposure to cancer-causing pesticides, metals, and chemicals
- ✔ Keep x-ray procedures to a minimum
- ✔ Avoid long-term use of hormone replacement therapy

Don't confuse recommendations on how to decrease the risk of developing cancer with a promise of preventing cancer. Scientists have defined many possible causes of cancer, but no one can say for sure what causes any individual to get cancer.

That said, all these health practices make for appropriate conversation with your doctor as you work out a wellness plan for your future.

Maybe you will integrate all these health practices into your life wholeheartedly. Maybe you will pick and choose what works for you. Maybe you will think about changing your lifestyle but not get around to it. Or maybe you will approach any changes suspiciously.

If you find yourself launching your new life tentatively, with more fear than hope, figuratively holding your breath to see what will happen next — if you are moving lightly through life, as though walking on eggs — we have a culinary suggestion:

Break those eggs! Stride right in and make omelets, eggs Benedict, crabmeat quiches, and scrambled eggs with fresh chives and feta cheese. Life, as many have said before, is a banquet. Eat up!

Chapter 19

Dealing with Recurrence: Here We Go Again

*Y*ou got it, you fought it, and you won. Then, when no one was looking — or maybe everyone was looking, and that's why you found it — cancer sneaked back in.

How unfair is that?

Almost everyone who has ever had cancer worries, or at least wonders, from time to time if the disease will recur. This chronic uneasiness, this lingering fear about recurrence, often is heightened on the anniversary of your first diagnosis or the night before you go for a scan or screening test. However, that fear can sweep through you just as easily under circumstances far more mundane. Even years later, the most rational mind can jump to the wrong conclusion when something unexpected triggers thoughts of recurrence.

Maybe what you've feared has happened, and your cancer is back. That means entering once again the culture of medical care — the world of tests and treatments, physical side effects, and emotional turmoil. Yet something is different. This time, you know what a formidable foe cancer can be, but you also know what you're made of. You know coping skills, ways to make treatments easier on yourself, and strategies to put in place to keep your spirits up and see you through.

You also know that you already beat this once, or you wouldn't be here now to face cancer again. Onward: It's time to take up arms again!

Defining Recurrence

Medically speaking, *recurrence* is the return of cancer some months or even years after you finish treatment for your original cancer. Cancer comes back because undetected cancer cells lurking somewhere in the body managed to avoid the head-to-toe mouthwash of chemotherapy, the relentless zapping of radiation, or the high precision of the surgeon's knife. At some point, these cells did what they do best — multiplied in preparation to make a new tumor or moved to a new spot in the body.

Before you panic and assume the worst, read this sentence: More and more often today, cancer is regarded as a chronic disease that may cause a series of flare-ups throughout your life.

With few exceptions, a recurrence is more serious than an original diagnosis of early-stage cancer. However, if you imagine that what automatically comes after a recurrence is a downhill slide into eternity, think again. You may find that new treatments have been developed since your first experience. Also, because you likely have been closely monitored, the tumor — if there is a tumor — may be smaller than the previous one and, therefore, easier to treat. There is more good news: In recent years, scientists have developed a number of new drugs that lessen the rigorous side effects that accompany treatments.

For many people, recurrence is not a death sentence because doctors can successfully treat many a recurrent cancer.

Recognizing signs of recurrence

Typically, recurrence brings with it symptoms that serve as warning signals to you and your doctor. When a symptom appears, tests and scans can confirm whether cancer has returned. Among these symptoms are

- A lump or swelling somewhere in the body
- Bone pain
- Chronic backaches
- Shortness of breath
- Declining appetite
- Unexpected weight loss
- Pain or weakness in arms or legs
- Chronic headaches

These symptoms are exactly the sort that you and your doctor have been watching for since your original diagnosis, and they are exactly the sort you want to report immediately.

Of course, anyone can experience one or more of these symptoms for reasons other than recurrence of cancer.

Getting up to speed on semantics

If you've got cancer again, is it new, or is it somehow connected to the previous diagnosis?

Cancer that recurs is not considered "new" cancer, even when it appears somewhere in your body away from the original site. When cancer comes back — regardless of where it is located — doctors typically find the same type of cells that were in the original tumor. That said, occasionally a person may be diagnosed with an all-new cancer with different kinds of cells. That's why biopsies are done: to see whether the cells look the same as the previous cancer cells or look different in some way.

Sometimes, cancer comes back at its original site. Sometimes, it reappears elsewhere. Typically, a recurrence is classified by where in the body it recurs. Here is a quick geography lesson:

- ✔ In a *local recurrence,* the cancer is in or very close to the same place as the original cancer.

- ✔ In a *regional recurrence,* the cancer is in the tissues or lymph nodes near the site of the original cancer.

- ✔ In a *distant recurrence,* the cancer has *metastasized,* or spread to organs or tissues beyond the site of the original cancer.

Early detection and early treatment are important factors in the outcome of most local recurrences. However, in some cancers, early detection and treatment do not provide the benefits you may hope for, especially in the case of a distant recurrence. That's because it's harder to fight cancer on several fronts at once after it has spread to multiple sites in the body.

Redefining Survivor

As time passed after your original cancer treatments ended, you may have come to think of yourself as a cancer survivor. And why not? The term is everywhere today, applied even to people just checking out of the hospital after cancer surgery, still woozy from the anesthesia. The National Coalition of Cancer Survivorship considers anyone with a history of cancer a "cancer survivor." In that sense, the term applies from the time of diagnosis to the end of life, regardless of the time span in between the two events.

Some people who have had cancer consider themselves survivors only after they deem themselves cured. However, *cured* is not a term you are likely to hear from your doctor, because doctors are acutely aware that cancer can recur at any time. Instead, doctors speak of people being *in remission,* which technically means that you inhabit a period of time when no cancer is detected in your body.

In remission may more accurately describe some people's medical situation, because microscopic cancer cells are not always immediately detectable. Does that mean it's dicey to think of yourself as a survivor while your doctor tells you that you are in remission? Of course not. Even if cancer recurs, you still can claim you are a survivor of the first encounter. Surviving — even thriving — is your goal the second time, as well.

Riding the Emotional Roller Coaster

At one time, the word on the street was that if your cancer did not recur within five years after the last treatment, you were safe for the rest of your life. Unfortunately, that simply isn't true. Cancer can recur at any time, even a decade or more after the first diagnosis. The longer a person is in remission, the less likely it is that the cancer will return or metastasize. However, "less likely" does not completely rule out a recurrence or even an entirely new cancer.

Some cancers have a reputation for recurring, but for others, the likelihood of recurrence is small. Maybe your doctor talked to you about this subject during your first experience, or maybe you opted not to hear the statistics.

Either way, when it's back, it's back.

Questioning everything

You may have all sorts of questions when you find out your cancer has returned:

- ✔ Did the chemotherapy miss some out-of-the-way cluster of cells?
- ✔ Did the radiation target need to be larger?
- ✔ Was the surgery not extensive enough?

✔ Did I choose the wrong doctor or hospital?

✔ Should I have asked for a second opinion the first time around?

✔ What if I had changed my diet after treatments ended, instead of falling back into my old eating habits?

✔ Was green tea the answer all along?

Yikes . . . these sorts of questions will get you nowhere but crazy!

While you're completely within your rights to ask these and all the other questions that come to mind, you'll most likely find that no one has definitive answers. As frustrating as that fact is, you can't let the unanswered questions rule your brain for long. Pondering these questions only uses up energy that you need to handle the recurrence.

That's not to say that you aren't entitled to take some time to absorb the news. When you hear that your cancer has come back, you may experience the same feelings as when you were first diagnosed. You remember the feelings. They include

✔ Shock

✔ Disbelief

✔ Fear

✔ Anxiety

✔ Depression

Don't be surprised if you also are angry, because once again your health is compromised and your life may be in danger. Yell at fate, yell at the test results, and yell at your body. No one will disagree that it's not fair to get cancer even once, much less twice.

But no matter how angry you get, try not to blame yourself or your medical team. You and your doctors made careful choices the first time around based on the information available. And just as you and your doctors did not cause your cancer the first time, you and your doctors did not cause the recurrence, either.

Moving on

Some people who survive cancer once actually spend time "practicing" for a recurrence by periodically allowing their minds to dwell on that possibility. Others think that's crazy and work hard to put plenty of emotional distance between themselves and the original diagnosis. Either way, hearing that the cancer is back may seem worse than hearing about it the first time, especially if you spend time trying to figure out who is to blame.

After you've let your emotions run their course, you need to find your resolve, take time to strengthen it, and focus on what's next. At this point, the only reasonable thing you can do is make plans for treatment a second time around.

Establishing a Treatment Plan

Not surprisingly, making a plan this time will not differ much from the first time. Your doctor will take these factors into account:

- ✔ Your age
- ✔ Your general health
- ✔ The type of cancer
- ✔ The location and size of the tumor

Of course, the doctor also will review when your original treatment took place, how well you handled that treatment, and how efficiently your body responded. This time, depending on all these factors, the doctor may recommend more aggressive treatment — or an entirely different treatment — than the first time around.

Understanding your options

Even though you've been down the treatment road before, make time to inform yourself (or refresh your memory) about your options. Among the possibilities are

- ✔ Surgery
- ✔ Radiation therapy
- ✔ Chemotherapy
- ✔ Hormone therapy
- ✔ Biologic therapy
- ✔ Bone marrow transplantation

Details on all these treatments are covered elsewhere in this book. Another option that may be available is a clinical trial (see Chapter 6). Your doctor also may encourage you to consider complementary therapies, which are covered in Chapter 14, to help reduce stress this time around.

When cancer recurs and is, for whatever reason, incurable, the doctor likely will switch goals from *curative* to *palliative*. What this means is that the doctor may recommend less aggressive therapies that induce fewer side effects and preserve quality of life. As we say earlier in this chapter, a recurrence usually is more serious than an original diagnosis of early-stage cancer. If your prognosis is not good, your doctor may speak to you about hospice care, which you can read about later in this chapter.

 No matter what your prognosis, discuss with your family and your doctor the risks, the side effects, and the impact of all available treatments on your quality of life. Also, ask your doctor about his treatment goals. And consider seeking a second opinion.

Making the most of past experiences

On days when you are absolutely certain that you do not want to go through cancer treatments again, and you are absolutely certain that you cannot manage it, consider this: Research shows that many people facing cancer a second time discover that they have significant advantages over people experiencing cancer for the first time. Here are just some of the things you have going for you:

- ✔ You already know what it's like to have cancer, so you have less fear.
- ✔ You already know individual doctors, nurses, medical technicians, and staff members at the clinic, hospital, or cancer center.
- ✔ You already know how the medical system works.
- ✔ You already know more medical terms than you had ever hoped to know.
- ✔ You already know how to navigate the health insurance system.
- ✔ You already know firsthand what to expect from cancer treatments in the way of side effects.
- ✔ You already know how to help alleviate those side effects.
- ✔ You already know how to ask for support from your family and friends, from support groups, from healthcare professionals, and from spiritual leaders.
- ✔ You already know how to help relieve stress by exercising, meditating, spending time with friends, and making time to laugh.

See? You have experience. Draw on that experience as you try to make the best of this unwanted occasion in your journey through life.

Setting treatment goals when a cure isn't possible

Now you know that when cancer recurs, many treatments are available, some of which have improved since your original diagnosis. You know that your firsthand experience gives you an edge, an advantage, over facing cancer the first time. And you know that in many instances, people triumph over a recurrence — sometimes more than one recurrence — and live for many years.

But what if you've been told you can't expect to live for many years? If cancer that returns a second or third time cannot be eradicated, you still have treatment options to consider. For instance, doctors can

✔ Stop or control the growth of a tumor

✔ Manage any pain you may have

✔ Help you minimize side effects

✔ Provide the highest quality of life for as long as possible

Many people with heart disease, diabetes, and even AIDS know how to live life to the fullest, savoring a high quality of life even with compromised health. So can you.

If your cancer is advanced, your doctor may recommend taking part in a clinical trial that would provide you with experimental therapy. One man we know with AIDS has been on numerous courses of experimental drugs for over ten years. We had hoped to interview him so we could share with you his refreshing philosophy of life, but he is busy serving as artistic director for a theater in the Midwest — and directing and acting in shows as well. Then again, now you know a little something about his philosophy of life.

Considering Unconventional Treatments

Lest you think that we advocate attempting any sort of experimental therapy that crosses your path, we need to make a distinction: Carefully monitored clinical trials are the medical profession's way of seeking innovative treatments — of moving medical care into the future. For information on complementary therapies and/or treatments that are currently under study, visit M.D. Anderson Cancer Center's Complementary/Integrative Medicine Education Resources (CIMER) Web site (www.mdanderson.org/departments/cimer) or the National Institutes of Health site for the National Center for Complementary and Alternative Medicine (www.nccam.nih.gov).

Why be cautious about trying an unconventional treatment? Because some experimental therapies available to you, such as herbs, dietary practices, and technological interventions, may have a better chance of relieving you of your money than your disease.

There's nothing wrong with trying these treatments as long as you know the risks and the limitations. For one thing, they haven't been tested in large clinical trials that would indicate whether they're truly helpful to people with cancer. For another, they aren't regulated the same way traditional cancer treatments are, so you likely won't be informed of any known or potential risks or side effects.

Among these unproven treatments are

- ✔ Macrobiotic diets: Eating programs restricted to whole grains and beans
- ✔ Coffee enemas: A detoxification regime
- ✔ Herbs and herbal teas: Products said to cure cancer or boost the immune system
- ✔ Laetrile: A plant compound found in the pits of some fruits and nuts
- ✔ Oxygenation treatments: The use of substances said to restore oxygen to tissues
- ✔ Negative ion therapy: Electromagnetic blasts of high-voltage electricity said to kill cancer

The appeal of some of these approaches is understandable. If conventional cancer treatments and regulated experimental drugs have failed to halt your cancer, you may figure that you have nothing to lose by trying unproven methods. Actually, you do have something to lose — money, of course, but also energy reserves and days in the sunshine that could be put to better use.

Unconventional cancer treatments may cause dangerous reactions in your body or may delay or interfere with other treatments you are undergoing. Be sure to speak with your doctor about any treatments that you are considering.

Facing the Future, Whatever Comes

Maybe your cancer cannot be eradicated. Maybe the disease this time is too advanced to respond to experimental drugs. What decisions are left to make? Perhaps the most important decision is how you'll spend your remaining time.

You may be the sort of person who wants every possible medical intervention right until the end, and if so, you likely will choose to spend your last days in a hospital that offers the best medical technology available. More power to you: That's the right choice for many people.

But when your doctors say they have done everything they can, and you are ready for them to do nothing more, you may want to consider *hospice* care — end-of-life care that can be provided in your home, the hospital, a nursing home, or a designated hospice facility.

Research reports that most Americans fear dying alone, dying out of control, and dying in pain. Hospice care addresses all three fears.

Finding comfort in hospice care

Hospice is compassionate end-of-life care for anyone expected to die within six months who chooses to let nature take its course. With hospice, a team of healthcare professionals comes to your home, your hospital, your nursing home, or a freestanding hospice to care for you and your family during this time.

The team, which coordinates care with your doctor, is skilled in symptom control; state-of-the-art pain management; and the delivery of tender, loving care. Typically, a hospice team includes

- A medical director
- A physician
- A social worker
- A nurse
- A home-health aide
- A spiritual adviser
- A bereavement counselor
- Trained volunteers

This team provides care, medical equipment, pain medication, and all medications related to your cancer. The goal is a quiet, natural death, absent of all "extraordinary measures" to cure or retard the cancer — a death that comes after you have reviewed the triumphs and joys of your life and said peaceful farewells to family members and friends.

Living "until you die"

Ciceley Saunders, a British nurse who returned to school to become a doctor, gets the credit for the modern hospice movement. As a nurse, Saunders was dissatisfied with how dying patients were cared for. At the age of 39, Saunders entered medical school and became a doctor. In 1967, she founded St. Christopher's Hospice in London. Saunders's pledge to those in hospice was this: "You matter to the last moment of your life, and we will do all we can not only to help you die peacefully, but to live until you die."

To this day, hospice is a popular choice throughout the world, but it is underused — and often misunderstood — in the United States. The National Hospice and Palliative Care Organization reports that some 775,000 patients nationwide used hospice for end-of-life care in 2001, a year when the National Center for Health Statistics recorded 2,416,425 deaths.

In 2003, some 3,300 hospice programs in the United States served some 950,000 people. People with cancer accounted for 49 percent of hospice patients. The median length of time spent in hospice per patient in 2003 was just 22 days, though people are eligible for hospice when the doctor estimates that they may live for only six months or less.

To find a hospice provider near you, see the Web site for the National Hospice and Palliative Care Organization at www.nhpco.org, or call 800-658-8898.

Debunking the myths of hospice

Hospice is underused in the United States (see the sidebar "Living 'until you die'"), and one reason is because of the persistence of several myths. For instance, many people wrongly believe that hospice is expensive. In truth, most hospice providers are Medicare-certified, and you bear few, if any, out-of-pocket expenses. Many insurance plans cover hospice or may be willing to convert a home-healthcare benefit to hospice care for younger people. Also, most hospice providers will make arrangements to care for people who have no insurance.

Another myth is the belief that hospice is only possible if you have family members to help care for you. In most cases, hospice providers work with other community programs to provide home care for people who have no family, or they can recommend locations where care is available.

Perhaps the oddest myth is that hospice care hastens death. That's simply not true. In some cases, people in hospice improve and are able to leave hospice care for a time. In fact, you are free to sign out of hospice care any time you choose, should you elect to give medical technology another chance.

Traveling on

If you do decide to consider hospice as you approach the end of your life, you may appreciate knowing that the word *hospice* comes from a medieval term for a travelers' way station. Today, hospice care is designed to assist "travelers" making their way through the necessary — and inevitable — separation from this life.

Chapter 20

Defining Yourself after Cancer: The New Normal

*F*or many people, cancer provides an emotional makeover. Here's why: Most people don't really believe that they are mortal, that the day will come when they no longer walk this earth. When you go through a life-threatening disease, you confront your mortality. You think about how much you would miss being alive, and you start paying more attention to everything that gives you pleasure right this minute, even if your hair hasn't all grown back after chemotherapy, your scar from surgery still itches, or your skin remains sensitive where you had radiation.

After cancer, more likely than not you suddenly understand from the inside out what really matters. You bring an entirely new perspective to such sayings as "Don't sweat the small stuff" and "Take time to smell the roses." Now you get that almost everything is "small stuff," and you make a mad dash for the nearest rosebush, ready to embrace petals, stems, thorns, and all.

Do you go from sad to happy, from depressed to gleeful, from pessimistic to optimistic all at once? Of course not. Emotional growth, the development of a new perspective, comes over time — two steps forward and one back, with some days bringing emotions that can only be described as mixed. In this chapter, you discover what to expect as this new you evolves and also how to protect yourself during the process.

Looking at Life Through New Eyes

Over time, as you change from seeing the word *cancer* in four-foot-high neon letters to seeing it in reasonable 10-point type like this, you begin to notice other changes as well. If you get a new boss at work, you don't panic about your ability to get along. When you run short of money one week, you figure there will be another paycheck soon enough. When your doctor tells you that you have a little arthritis in your knees, you smile and say you can manage that.

Having cancer gives you a new perspective on life. Multi-taskers learn to appreciate the concept of doing one thing at a time, and doing it well. People enamored of the "all work and no play" philosophy of life come to embrace balance. Even Type A sorts calm down, chill out, and realize they don't have to be in charge of the world this week — or maybe even for the rest of the month. This new perspective gives you an edge you may previously have been missing, and even years after treatments end, you will be able to call on the calm certainty that no matter what happens, you can handle it. "Hey," you will say to yourself and anyone within earshot, "it's not cancer." Then you will start resolving whatever "it" is.

At some point, you may go so far as to say that cancer changed your life for the better. If you do, you won't be alone in that regard. In one recent study, as many as 83 percent of women questioned one year after treatment reported at least one benefit from having breast cancer.

Reaping the benefits

Here are some of the benefits that some cancer survivors report after spending time with this life-threatening disease:

- ✔ Appreciation for each new day
- ✔ Realignment of priorities at home and work
- ✔ Heightened awareness of each sunrise and sunset
- ✔ Commitment to a more balanced life
- ✔ Pride in overcoming adversity
- ✔ Increased sense of personal power
- ✔ Decrease in timidity or shyness

✔ Higher emphasis on personal health

✔ Bolder attitude about trying new things

✔ Connectedness with other cancer survivors

✔ Willingness to accept less than perfection from yourself and others

Perhaps the most important question you can ask yourself when you are diagnosed is not, "Why me?" but "What can I learn from this?"

Now you know.

Getting a physical boost from positive thinking?

Right this minute, studies are in progress to determine whether looking for the good in a bad experience helps boost the immune system. Some research has indicated that when you look for the proverbial silver lining, your immune system may grow stronger. The jury is still out on this prospect — and it may be out for years, as more studies are conducted — but anyone who has been up as well as down will tell you that being happy takes less energy than being sad.

That's not to say that you do yourself great harm by expressing negative feelings. Acknowledging sadness, fatigue, or even fear is often the first important step in getting help if you need it. (See Chapters 10 and 13 for information on how to recognize depression and how to get help.) Besides, it's better to admit that you're down in the dumps sometimes than to wear yourself out trying to be positive all the time.

However, if you're stressed more often than not, make it a priority to spend some time working to reduce your stress so your attitude — and possibly the efficiency of your immune system — can improve. The National Cancer Institute recommends some of the following ways to reduce stress, and we've added a few of our own:

✔ Begin an exercise program.

✔ Take up dancing or movement.

✔ Consider joining a support group.

✔ Enroll in music or art classes.

✔ Talk to a member of the clergy or a spiritual advisor.

> ✔ Keep a journal.
>
> ✔ Provide encouragement for a friend starting cancer treatments.
>
> ✔ Set some new goals for yourself.
>
> ✔ Decide to speak positively about your experience with cancer.

We have more to say on that last one.

Making Semantic Decisions

Somewhere every day, a cancer survivor talking to a group, large or small, begins the speech with, "Thank you! I'm happy to be here. But then, people who have been through cancer are happy to be anywhere."

Powerful words, those. Are they true? Well, you get to decide what to say about how well or how poorly you are doing after cancer treatments or how happy you are to be here. When someone asks how you are, you choose which words to use. You can grin and reply that you are just fine, or you can regale the questioner with a list of everything that could be better. (In fairness, even people who have never had cancer sometimes keep such a list at the ready just in case someone asks about their health.)

If you believe that it is up to you to make the most of any "borrowed time" you are granted after a diagnosis of cancer, most likely you will choose positive words to describe your health and circumstances.

Allowing for Negativity

Let's be honest: Not every cancer survivor believes that he is better off than before cancer. A recent study reported in the *Journal of the National Cancer Institute* shows that cancer survivors "have poorer health, lose more days from work and have a generally lower quality of life than people who have never had the disease." Keep in mind that the study emphasizes physical health, and as we explain in Chapter 18, lingering side effects are common months or even years after cancer treatments end.

What if that study had asked cancer survivors whether they are glad to be alive?

We're not trying to say that you won't be sad or bitter from time to time about any losses you may have suffered as a result of having cancer, or about your current level of physical function. But most people are glad to still be in the game. The thing about games (and we're talking baseball here) is that sometimes you strike out, and sometimes you hit a home run. Sometimes, you save the game with a dramatic catch in the outfield, and sometimes you are stuck on the bench. Sometimes, you are even on the disabled list. Sometimes, of course, you lose, but sometimes you win.

The uncertainty of the game of life may be enough at times to make you want to pick up your ball and glove and go home. But then what?

Not playing at all isn't any fun. Maybe you're better off in the game after all, even though neither you nor anybody else gets any guarantees about the outcome.

Finding Inspiration in Amazing Recoveries

If you're feeling down about your physical limitations, consider the stories of some professional athletes who took a curve ball (cancer, that is) and came back into the game. These athletes were superlative examples of strength, stamina, and style in their particular arena, award-winning players who personified the peak of physical fitness. They then underwent surgery, chemotherapy, and radiation, and later they asked themselves to get back in the game, on the field, on the bike, in the rink . . . back to a peak level of fitness. And they did it.

If you're like most people who have been treated for cancer, you probably just want to get back to the office or the family or the serenity that normal, day-to-day living can offer. Don't you feel relieved already, knowing that you aren't expecting yourself to resume hitting home runs in the major leagues?

That's what baseball player Eric Davis did. Davis was diagnosed with colon cancer in May of 1997, and he had surgery the following month. Late that September, Davis was back playing with the Baltimore Orioles, though he was still taking chemotherapy treatments. With two days left in the season, Davis hit a home run deep into the stands in left center. In his autobiography, *Born to Play* (Signet), Davis writes:

> *"The fact that I was in that uniform, out there competing, made the fans see another side of me and allowed them to learn something about recovering from cancer that maybe they thought they'd never see or learn. They embraced a lot of things about my recovery that were there in them, too — that a man or a woman can come back from cancer and not just exist, but produce at the same level — at a higher level."*

Lance Armstrong is a "higher level" survivor. The professional cyclist was diagnosed with testicular cancer that had spread to his lungs, abdomen, and brain. Nonetheless, after grueling surgery and treatment in 1996, three years later Armstrong won the equally grueling Tour de France, which covers 2,290 miles and takes three weeks to finish. To date, Armstrong has won that race six times! In his biography, *It's Not About the Bike: My Journey Back to Life* (Berkley Publishing Group), Armstrong writes, "I'm not a victim. I'm a survivor."

Scott Hamilton, the Olympic skater, was diagnosed with testicular cancer in 1997. He writes about his experience in his book *Landing It: My Life On and Off the Ice* (Pinnacle Books). Four months after surgery, Hamilton took his first tentative steps back onto the ice. Two months later, he performed for 15,000 people. At the end of that show, Hamilton grabbed a microphone and declared, "I WIN."

Winning is relative after cancer. Even if you don't ask yourself to exceed your former level of physical fitness, you can win under the terms of the new "normal."

Looking at Time Differently

"People think time is money," says oncologist and author Dr. Bernie Siegel. "It's not. Time is everything." After cancer, in most cases, you understand that fact, and you want to make the most of your time. Some people consider that to be the primary lesson that cancer teaches.

Hearing the wakeup call

In William Elliott's book *Tying Rocks to Clouds* (Image), meditation teacher Jack Kornfeld considers the importance of time:

> *"We often put off what we know, thinking our lives will last forever, or very long. Very long is not forever. Then all of a sudden we find someone near us dies or we get sick and realize, Whoa, I better live in ways that I haven't because I thought I had time."*

Droning along in a ho-hum job? Cancer will teach you that it's later than you think — that today is the perfect day to change your life. You learn that working for a living matters, but not nearly as much as working on a life, and you adjust your schedule accordingly. Maybe you decide to stick to an eight-hour day, giving up that unpaid overtime, or you figure out how to make the family budget work if you go into the office only four days a week. Maybe, on some sunny, beautiful Tuesday morning, you play hooky. Did the office get along without you when you were out sick after cancer surgery? Then they can manage if you miss a Tuesday.

You likely will be more careful during your leisure hours, as well. Sitting in a self-help seminar that strikes you as too precious, watching a movie that bores you, or wasting time surfing the Web? After cancer, you have a built-in "life is too short" alarm, and when it goes off after 45 minutes at that seminar, that movie, or your desk, you get up and walk away. Use the time to take a walk, have a cup of coffee or tea on your deck, or look through seed catalogues and plan your garden. Are you the industrious sort who never used vacation time that you had coming? Bring on those travel brochures! Or just pile into the car with the kids and go check out the attractions in a neighboring state. Make the most of the time you have.

After cancer, you learn to look at time differently. And sooner rather than later, you find yourself shuddering inwardly when you overhear someone say they are "just killing time."

Living in gratitude

Some people differentiate between what cancer teaches them and what they learn from surviving. In 2004, political columnist Molly Ivins told coauthor Patricia that Ivins had had a recurrence after first being treated successfully for breast cancer in 1999. "Having cancer is not a lovely experience, and I gained no great insight from it," Ivins said. "However, afterward, like every survivor, I was incredibly grateful."

That gratitude inspired Ivins to return to Paris for a visit after a 35-year absence, and she began taking piano lessons — a lifelong dream — when approaching her 60th birthday. Surviving, rather than the cancer itself, may be what makes you more aware of the gift of time.

Spending time on yourself

You have been given an opportunity to consider parceling out your time differently. If you have spent much of your life making others happy or doing only what everyone else has expected, now is the time to recognize your own worth and spend some time making yourself happy. What should you do first? Anything goes — here are some ideas to get you thinking:

- Read a book on seashells or the different species of cacti.
- Plant an herb garden.
- Join a local museum and take a tour.
- Help out at your grandchild's school.
- Research your family history.
- Settle in for a nap on the couch with the cat.
- Take an art class or learn a new language.
- Take a neighbor's child to the zoo or the park.
- Volunteer at the cancer education center at a nearby hospital.

In other words, after cancer, you have the perfect excuse to reconsider everything you have been doing, drop what is no longer useful, and create a new "normal" for yourself.

If the very thought of all this restructuring makes you tired, remember that you don't have to make every change in the first week. Still, after some time breathing deeper and smiling at all that is around you, you are more likely to experiment with new attitudes, new points of view, new perspectives — even new verbs.

A gift of new beginnings

In January 1997, your coauthor Patricia made a two-week trip to Egypt on a tour led by a fifth-generation Egyptologist. She went, she says, "because during chemotherapy, I had dreamed I was standing outside the Great Pyramid at Giza. I also went because a year earlier, I couldn't, and now I could." Here is her story:

I knew before I went to Egypt that scarab jewelry was popular, but I didn't know why. While touring the tomb of Nefertari in the Valley of the Queens, our guide told us that the scarab is the symbol of new beginnings. "New beginnings! That's why I'm here in Egypt," I thought to myself. I decided right then to buy a scarab souvenir of some sort.

I didn't have to. After the tour of the tombs, we headed back to the bus. The driver had brought along his 11-year-old son, who sat across from me. Earlier in the day, I had noticed the boy watching me scan the sky for birds with my binoculars. Before our group left the bus to tour the tombs, I had handed the binoculars to the boy and told him to enjoy himself. Upon my return, he thanked me and gave them back. Then, shyly, he placed something on the seat next to me.

It was a small alabaster carving of a scarab. "This is for you," he said.

Charlotte Perkins Gilman, a writer and lecturer who lived from 1860 to 1935, once declared that life is a verb. Yet most of us meander along treating life as a common noun, or maybe even as a wimpy adjective, until some specific event, such as cancer, jolts us out of our daydreams and smack into the present moment. That transformation allows us to recognize that finishing cancer treatments is a perfect time for beginning anew.

Protecting Yourself Emotionally

So now you're up to speed on this issue of looking at time differently after cancer and hearing the wake-up call loud and clear. That alone makes you less vulnerable to the uncertainty that comes when you finish cancer treatments. In Chapter 18, we talk about the fear of recurrence, and Chapter 19 is all about recurrence itself. One of the best ways to fend off this very normal fear — as well as the fear that every sinus infection, strained muscle, and headache means the cancer is back — is to learn to protect yourself emotionally.

Looking out for number one

Frankly, no protective measure is too small when it comes to maintaining emotional equilibrium in the early weeks and months after treatments end. Here are some practical suggestions to help you do just that:

- **Turn the page.** Say you're minding your own business, reading the weekend newspaper, or maybe you're looking through a magazine at the dentist's office. You turn the page, and there you find an article about the horrors of cancer, with shocking color photos of people in the last stages of the disease. Your heart beats faster and your pulse races. You have one sure way to save yourself unwanted anxiety — turn the page again.

- **Change the channel.** You're taking it easy one evening after dinner, surfing the channels on your television set. By coincidence, you pause on one of those medical shows, and you see a character dying of cancer, surrounded by next of kin. Grab the remote and move on.

- **Walk out of the movie.** In your former life, maybe you enjoyed those tear-jerker movies that required a purse full of tissues before the film ended, usually in the death of one of the leading actors. If by some well-intentioned set of circumstances you find yourself in one of those movies now, get up and leave. See if an upbeat Disney picture or a romantic comedy is showing in the theater next door.

✔ **Stop the storyteller.** Here you are, a cancer survivor eager to move on, to embrace the new beginnings you have fashioned for yourself. You run into an acquaintance you haven't seen in some time who first tells you that you're looking swell and then starts in on a painful story about Aunt Louise or Uncle Mac who has the same kind of cancer and just entered hospice care. Put your hand on this person's shoulder, remark how hard it all must be for the family, and say you really must run. Then get a move on. Do not listen to the story.

You owe no one any apologies for choosing not to wallow in the past, in sadness, or in fear.

Making friends with lingering fear

President Franklin Delano Roosevelt told us that we have nothing to fear but fear itself. Frankly, after cancer there is no point in being afraid of fear. Respecting fear and the kind of stress it can cause is sensible, but you have an opportunity now to forge a different kind of relationship as well.

You may want to consider making friends with fear by acknowledging its power. Think about it this way: In the winter, you try to protect yourself from catching the flu by staying away from sick people, keeping your hands away from your face, and washing your hands often with warm water and plenty of antibacterial soap. You know about the threat of flu, and you take necessary precautions in the hope of avoiding it.

You can treat fear the same way. Acknowledge the possibility that it can hurt you, and then work to protect yourself. For starters, go back and reread the previous section.

Defining Your Boundaries at Home and Work

As you sort out your new normal and realign your world now that cancer is part of your past, you also will notice changes in some of your relationships. In Chapter 2, we advise that you may want to expect the unexpected regarding the news of your diagnosis. Some people may have trouble handling the news and turn to you for help. Some won't know what to say or do and may just disappear from your life for a while. The same is true at this point.

Family members who were 100 percent supportive during your treatments may assume that now you are ready to go back to "the way things were." They may expect you to resume all the household duties and chores you had before your diagnosis, and the sooner the better. You may be willing but realize that your body isn't ready. Maybe you are not willing — you like the new division of labor at your house so well that you want to leave it in place from now on. Or, maybe a pristine house and carefully trimmed lawn don't seem as important to you now as they once did.

A similar situation may come up at work. More likely than not, your level of productivity will rise over the next few months as you continue to recover from the treatments. However, maybe your boss is impatient, or maybe you've decided to seek a less stressful or physically demanding position, either in your current workplace or elsewhere.

How do you handle these situations? Here are some tips:

- ✔ Explain that recovery is a gradual process.
- ✔ Speak frankly about what you think you can do, can't do, and choose not to do.
- ✔ Request any changes that would make your home life or your work environment better for you.

 Ask your doctor for help explaining your situation to family members or work colleagues. Also, if you think you are being discriminated against at work in any way, talk to a manager or union representative. If you must, call the local bar association for names of lawyers who handle employment discrimination cases.

Lightening Up

Laughter, as the saying goes, is the best medicine. In Chapter 2, we explain the importance of keeping your sense of humor during treatments. After treatments have ended is no time to get serious. In fact, one of the best things you can do for yourself as you define your new normal is spend more time with people who make you laugh.

Remember that buddy who crashed one of your pity parties early on and helped you laugh at your own sense of melodrama? After your hair fell out, did your college-age son comment on your striking resemblance to Jean-Luc

Picard on *Star Trek*? What about the friend who went wig shopping with you and hugged you, laughing, as she announced that your new "fake" hair looked better than your real hair? Is there someone in your life who took a book on cancer that upset you, threw it in the street, and then drove over it?

Find these people — and more like them. Embrace them and laugh with them all as you bask in the renewed joy of living.

Part VII
The Part of Tens

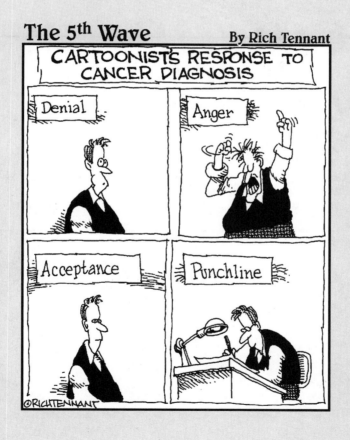

In this part . . .

Looking for talking points, such as easy-to-read lists recounting myths about cancer or specific things people can do to help you? Here you are! We've also come up with ten things beyond your control (which you can scratch off your list of worries), as well as ten gifts from cancer — unexpected benefits that make your new "normal" more rewarding. Lastly, we direct you to ten sources of additional information about cancer treatments.

Chapter 21

Ten Myths about Cancer

Some myths are delightful, like the one about the pink dolphins said to emerge from Peruvian rivers at night, turn into red-haired people, and go dancing. (They wear hats to hide their blowholes.) Other myths are frightening and can be dangerous to your sense of well-being, especially when you're being treated for cancer.

Sometimes, people who think they know everything pass on knowledge that is flawed, information that is outdated, and rumors that are simply false. In this chapter, we look at ten all-too-common misconceptions about cancer and set the record straight.

Myth #1: When You Get Cancer, You Die

That's just not so. The National Cancer Institute and the Centers for Disease Control and Prevention reported in 2004 that the number of people living with cancer in the United States increased from 3 million in 1971 to 9.8 million in 2001.

"In the absence of other competing causes of death," reads a summary of the report, "an estimated 64 percent of adults whose cancer was diagnosed during 1995 through 2000 could expect to be alive five years after diagnosis."

The health agencies have a stated objective that calls for increasing to 70 percent the proportion of cancer patients who are living more than five years after diagnosis. They hope to achieve this goal among adults by 2010, if more adults with cancer are willing to participate in clinical research trials. (The goal has already been met among children.)

That said, some people do die of cancer. The rest of us die of other causes.

Myth #2: If the Cancer Doesn't Kill You, the Treatments Will

No doubt about it, chemotherapy and radiation — standard treatments for most people with cancer — are rough. We explain these treatments in detail in Chapters 4 and 5. In Chapters 8 and 12, we go along with you (in the virtual sense) to your first appointment for each, and then we tell you everything you need to know about side effects in Chapters 10, 11, and 13.

If you have any doubt about the effectiveness of these treatments, go back and read Myth #1.

Research continues both on how to make chemotherapy and radiation more effective and on how to make the side effects easier to bear.

Myth #3: Cancer Treatments Are One-Size-Fits-All

Chemotherapy and radiation are standard cancer treatments. However, there are many combinations of chemotherapy drugs and several delivery systems, just as there are several kinds of radiation therapy. Your treatment plan is designed specifically for you, taking many personal factors (and facts about your particular cancer) into consideration.

You won't receive exactly the same cancer treatments as your brother-in-law, your aunt, your neighbor, or your co-worker. Your doctors will develop a custom treatment plan for you.

Myth #4: You Can't Work while You're Having Cancer Treatments

Many, many people not only *can* continue to work during cancer treatments — they *do*. Will you do your best work while coping with side effects? Maybe not, but in many cases you can put in a full day's work for a full day's pay throughout your treatments.

Myth #5: It Takes Forever to Get Over Cancer Treatments

It doesn't, really, though you may get weary waiting for your hair to grow back, your radiated skin to heal, your appetite to return, or your energy level to climb back to normal. Months from now, when you are enjoying better health, you will look back and realize that your recovery did take time — but not forever.

 That said, be sure to keep your boss in the loop about your treatments and be honest about how you're handling the side effects. In some instances, employees going through cancer treatments can request lighter duty for a few months or work fewer hours. But we can't promise what your situation will bring: Jobs, like cancer treatments, are not one-size-fits-all.

Myth #6: It's Your Fault You Got Cancer

No, it isn't. In Chapter 2, we tell you that cancer originates at the cellular level for reasons that are not entirely understood. Scientists have identified risk factors for cancer — among them smoking, drinking too much alcohol, eating an unhealthy diet, and exposing unprotected skin to the sun's rays. Still, not everybody who willfully practices these behaviors gets cancer. Cancer also cannot be blamed on a personality flaw, stress over the death of a loved one, a lapse in religious practices, or voting for the wrong candidate.

Furthermore, you did not get cancer because of stress in your life. And if someone tells you that in order to be cured of cancer you are required to banish all stress from your life, that's not true either. Both are commonly held beliefs, though there is little evidence to support either one.

If you take one thing away from this chapter, take this: It's not your fault.

Myth #7: The Medical Community Suppresses Alternative Healing Methods

Some vendors of nonregulated dietary supplements that claim to cure cancer insist that the healthcare industry, working hand in hand with the government, suppresses the scientific truth about such products because the profit margin is smaller than from sales of standard anticancer drugs.

That's a fine conspiracy theory, but it isn't true. In 1992, the U.S. government established the National Center for Complementary and Alternative Medicine, which is "dedicated to exploring complementary and alternative healing practices in the context of rigorous science." Medical researchers conduct studies of traditional and indigenous medicine (such as Native American medicine, Ayurvedic medicine, and traditional Chinese medicine), as well as studies of plant-based supplements. Curious about the results? See the Web site www.nccam.nih.gov.

Myth #8: Now Your Family Will All Get Cancer

Plenty of people who get cancer do not have a family history of the disease. However, cancer in the family does typically lead to an increased risk of the disease in successive generations. (Note that a risk is not a guarantee — remember that not everyone who smokes gets cancer either.)

Here's the good news: Knowing about the increased risk often prompts family members to be vigilant about getting the necessary screening tests, so if they do develop cancer, it can be caught early and treated before much damage is done.

Myth #9: Cancer Always Comes Back

"Always" is one of those gambling words, like "never." After you are diagnosed with cancer and have completed your treatments, your doctor may offer a *prognosis,* or prediction, regarding the likelihood of recurrence. She may be right — or wrong.

Cancer does not always come back, but if it does, take heart (and take a look at Chapter 19, where we talk about recurrence). Today, doctors can success-fully treat many recurrent cancers.

Myth #10: Nothing Is Ever the Same after Cancer

Okay, this myth has a lot of truth to it. But then, nothing is ever the same after your first kiss, or the birth of your first child, or your 40th birthday, or your first trip to Venice. Frankly, nothing is ever the same — ever — whether you get cancer or not.

Some people say that change is good. You may or may not agree, but this we know to be true: Change is inevitable.

Chapter 22

Ten Ways for Family and Friends to Help You

*I*f you've read other chapters of this book, you already know how important it is to put together a support team to help you get through cancer treatments. In terms of emotional support, family members and friends typically serve as the lead dogs, so to speak.

In this chapter, you find specific ways they can help you — suggestions that go above and beyond driving you to chemotherapy or picking up your dry cleaning. Those are important tasks, too, but here are the biggies.

Acknowledging That You Have Cancer

Make sure that the people you love are sitting down when you tell them, because the announcement that you have cancer literally can bowl some people over. Allow your family members and friends a few minutes of denial, anger, or fear — whatever they need to work through. And then, when the attention turns back to you, they need to acknowledge that you have a life-threatening disease, and they need to tell you they will do whatever they can to help.

Some individuals may not be able to provide the type of support you're looking for. That's fine — honestly. Try not to blame anyone or cut anyone out of your life because they can't support you at this difficult time. Some good people simply can't handle the "C" word. That doesn't mean they can't be there for you when you need them at another time of your life.

However, don't put anybody on your support team who needs to be propped up, because you're going to be too busy.

Giving You Time to Accept the Diagnosis

Everybody processes trouble differently. If you need to spend some time in denial or feeling angry at life or terrified of death, take it. Family and friends must let you set the pace on this one and follow your lead — at least to your face. If they express concerns later, speaking among themselves, that's fine. But it isn't fine to expect you to operate on anyone else's emotional timetable.

The same is true when you have recurring bouts of sadness or depression about your cancer in the coming months. It's unrealistic for anyone to expect you to face up to your diagnosis once at the beginning and then move forward, calm and confident ever after. However, someone — or several someones — may have that expectation.

You have the disease, you go for treatments, and you get to set any timetable that works for you regarding emotional adjustments. These things take time, and no one who has not had cancer can fully understand just how big an adjustment is required.

Holding You While You Cry

This task isn't an easy one, so choose one or two people you trust completely. Put on your game face for everybody else, but make it clear that sometimes, you just need to be held while you cry. Don't underestimate the importance of this kind and loving gesture throughout treatments. Crying alone is far less satisfying — and besides, being held is reassuring.

These private moments when you cry on the shoulder of a loved one help make up for the many appearances you must make in public wearing a brave mask. Neither posture is false. Dealing with cancer seems to require brave moments and moments of self-pity as well — not to mention a full range of moods in between!

Making You Laugh

Put all the funny people in your life — the great wits, the jokesters, the folks who do "big room" material at every opportunity — on notice that you need to be entertained, and often. Ask these people to watch funny movies with you or write family-based song parodies for you or — in the case of little ones — tell you every joke they hear in the third grade classroom.

Make sure your schedule is booked with more time for laughing than crying.

Seeking Help Coping from Someone Else

On those occasions when a family member or friend seems overwhelmed by helping to take care of you, acknowledge their months in service, put them on voluntary leave, and gently insist that they find somebody — anybody but you — to help them cope with the sometimes exhausting experience of belonging to a support team.

In other words, don't take on the burden right now of helping others cope as they help you. With any luck, you'll have other family members or friends who can step in where needed. Don't wait for them to notice the need: Make the call, and simply explain that you think a person with a starring role in your cancer drama needs an understudy to fill in for a while.

Asking for Specific Ways to Help You

Good friends ask how they can help. Best friends rattle off a list of possible acts that will save you time, energy, and worry. If you have either one on your support team, count your blessings.

Keep in mind that when someone asks to help, your requests don't always have to be logical. Maybe you and your sore throat are craving hazelnut gelato that's sold at only one store in town, which is 30 miles from your house. Don't be afraid to ask — you may be surprised how willing your friends are to accommodate!

Carrying Out Your Requests

Occasionally, a friend will call to say that he intends to bring over supper "sometime next week" or to get two tickets to the new movie you mentioned wanting to see. A well-meaning friend makes the call. A real friend follows through.

Sometimes people go astray when it comes to actually helping — they mean well, but they don't follow up. If you have this experience, prompt the person to get back in the game. Being available for generic "help" is not the same as actually helping.

Offering What You Are Reluctant to Ask For

You may hesitate to ask for certain kinds of help, perhaps because doing so would involve bringing up a touchy subject. Ideally, you want to have at least one person on your support team who knows you so well that he or she anticipates what you need and helps you get it even when you don't ask.

For example, if your sister knows that you don't have a will, knows that you are worried about that fact (especially right now), but also knows that you think talking about it will upset her, we hope your sister boldly brings up the subject and drives you to the lawyer's office. The same goes for drawing up an advance directive for healthcare (also known as a "living will") and a power of attorney document for health decisions. Both are extremely important documents.

Talking openly about sensitive subjects often reduces some of the anxiety for all concerned.

On the other hand, maybe you just wish that someone would offer to clean out the cat's litter box once a week. Good luck with that!

Helping to Protect You

During cancer treatments, you are at risk for infection. Members of your support team need to prohibit anyone with a nasty cold or respiratory infection from coming near you during particularly vulnerable times. You also are at risk for scaring yourself by reading too many cancer horror stories online or devoting too much time to the obituary section of the newspaper, counting up the deaths each day from cancer.

Observant family members and friends can help protect you from others — and from yourself. Accept this assistance with some degree of grace and gratitude, even if you are the one in the family known for protecting others.

Celebrating with You

As you go through treatments, acknowledge every meaningful landmark. Whether the occasion is marked by dinner out with a dozen friends or just a jubilant phone call, people who care about you will care enough to notice that you've reached the halfway point in radiation therapy or that you've successfully completed your first — or fourth, or last — round of chemotherapy. Cheering you on is just one more task for the team, and celebrating does everybody good.

It takes a village to get you through treatments. When your energy is back, have the gang over — invite the doctors, too — for a "thank you" party.

Chapter 23

Ten Things Beyond Your Control

In This Chapter

▶ Accepting — and admitting — your diagnosis

▶ Letting yourself rest

▶ Accepting help from one and all

*T*he good thing about situations beyond your control is that you don't have to spend time worrying about them. After all, if you have no control over the situation, what's the point?

Control is a big issue when you are going through cancer treatments. You quickly learn that in many instances, your role is simply to show up and allow things to be done to you. That passivity requires quite an adjustment for many of us, but the sooner you give in, the sooner you can move on to those matters that you do control.

In this chapter, we enumerate some worries that you may dispense with immediately.

Turning Back the Clock

It's too late not to get cancer, no matter how much you would prefer to cancel the diagnosis. Also, you can forget about signing up for special cancer insurance. (You don't know irony until you get an advertisement in the mail for that insurance on a day when you've just returned from radiation therapy.)

For better or worse, you are spending part of your life dealing with cancer. But remember, what's going on now will not go on forever. It may sound trite, but these words of wisdom are true: This too shall pass.

Keeping the Diagnosis a Secret

No matter how much you wish that the world would not find out about your diagnosis and treatments, somehow, word will get out. Certainly, you can choose whom to tell personally, and you can ask friends and co-workers not to talk about it, but these stories always have a way of spreading.

One thing you can do, should you be a private person, is control *how much* information goes out. Usually, people in this situation tell close family members and friends a great deal and then edit the information considerably for others. For many people, the expurgated version is plenty, as the primary concern may simply be how you are doing — not necessarily how you are doing it.

In other words, you don't have to tell everybody everything every time you are questioned. Hey, matters could be worse. We know a man who had extensive hair transplants that he rigorously declined to discuss, so everyone simply assumed that his head looked the way it did because of a critical illness.

Encountering an Alien Culture

For some reason, most of us (even rabid fans of the show *ER*) usually don't think about hospitals or the people in them, even when we drive by hospitals almost every day. The world inside a hospital, the world of medical professionals and medical treatments, is huge, complex, and completely different from the world of people who enjoy good health. The culture of illness is alien — it is different, though not in a negative way, because the people who inhabit that culture generally are caring professionals.

You would do well to embrace this alien culture during the time that you are part of it. Don't worry so much about how you got there as about how soon you can get back to your world.

Making New Friends

Maybe you don't think that you need or want any new friends, and maybe you have made up your mind not to go out of your way to meet new people while going through cancer treatments. Fine. Still, one day you may find yourself starting up a conversation with the person sitting next to you in the chemo infusion lounge or in the waiting room at radiation therapy.

Typically, people going through similar experiences make good compatriots, so don't worry if you end up breaking your own rule. Besides, you may pick up some helpful tips on handling side effects from someone who knows tricks you have yet to learn.

Experiencing Mood Swings

One minute, you're angry; the next, you're sad. An hour from now you may be philosophical and contemplative. All these emotions — and just about any others that you care to name — are completely normal for this time in your life. You are not crazy; you simply are handling a disturbing diagnosis and making a lot of important decisions that will affect the rest of your life. Worry about those decisions, if you must, but don't worry about occasional periods of emotional instability.

Facing Your Own Mortality

You've heard people start sentences with, "If I die. . . ." Frankly, this is wishful thinking, and it would be more correct to say, "When I die. . . ." Here's the thing about dying: It's very scary and extremely unsettling to think about it in personal terms. Before cancer, many people do not think about it at all. After cancer, when you have been made aware that you do not get to live forever, you may start to live differently — in a way that guarantees you get the most out of every moment.

If you make positive changes as a result of having cancer, you won't waste time worrying about dying because you will be busy living.

Suffering Power Outages

The first few times that you overextend yourself or ask too much of yourself physically, your body likely will demand that you head off to bed to recover. That may seem startling, especially if you're a person who's used to getting a lot done every day.

Our best advice: Don't worry about it. Cancer treatments cause fatigue, period. You're going to have less energy right now than you usually do. Accept that fact — even embrace it. And as you drift off to sleep, comfort yourself with the knowledge that what is true for now will not be true forever. Meanwhile, honor the needs of your body.

Missing Some Good Times

The naps that you likely will need may cause you to miss some get-togethers, some special events, and even some entire holidays. Sleep on. After your treatments end, you will have plenty of opportunities to have good times with family and friends.

Choosing the Texture of Your New Hair

You say that you've always had straight hair, and you want it to grow in curly after chemotherapy? Forget about it. Sure, your hair *may* come in completely different — then again, it may not. As with so many issues in life, you don't get to choose. You didn't get to choose what you had before, either, and somehow you made do. Besides, there is something to be said just for having hair again, curly or straight.

Receiving Help from Many Sources

Most people who go through cancer later report how astonished they are at how many people — some of them strangers — come forward to help in countless ways. Where do these people come from? Your extended family, your friends, your neighbors, your co-workers, people you worship with, and sometimes people you met once and will never see again all will commit unexpected acts of kindness directed at you as you go through this challenging time.

Don't worry: None of them expect thank-you notes. You can pay back these favors down the road by committing unexpected acts of kindness of your own to help others going through cancer.

Chapter 24

Ten Ways Life Will Be Better after Cancer

*T*en is only a smattering of the many ways that cancer may change your life for the better. Some of the changes are obvious early on; others may be subtle and take a while to develop. Some changes may present themselves as options — changes that you may decide to accept or reject.

In any case, cancer, a life-threatening disease, most often also is a life-changing experience. In this chapter, we explain why.

Cancer Goes Away

One obvious change, and an outstanding one at that, is that after cancer, your doctors will tell you that for now — and maybe forever — you no longer have cancer. What a grand and glorious day that is! It's been a long journey, and a celebration is in order.

Treatments End

Though you see your doctors from time to time and undergo the occasional screening test, after cancer you no longer have to endure treatments or put up with their side effects. After cancer, life is all about slowly getting better every day, gaining back strength and energy, and feeling more like yourself as each day passes.

At one time, your calendar was filled with treatment dates and follow-up appointments. No more. Now, you can use your calendar for other things:

- Pencil in lunch dates.
- Schedule an appointment to tour a new fitness center near you.
- Sign up to volunteer one morning a week at a local cancer education center.
- Meet with a person planning to run for political office.
- Sign up to accompany your grandchild's class field trip.

Fill other deliciously empty dates on the calendar with plans to spend time on yourself at the zoo, botanical garden, library, or day spa.

Fear Recedes

After cancer, your fear of the disease lessens bit by bit. As the months go by, you think less and less often about the experience of having cancer. Whole days, and then weeks, go by when you don't think about it at all.

In years to come — and we have this on good authority, straight from long-time survivors — you may even forget, unless reminded, that you ever had cancer. Imagine that!

A Sense of Adventure Grows

Just about the time your hair grows back, you may also grow a sense of daring, a wild side. You may head for Florida to ride on an airboat, make reservations at a really nice restaurant, buy two cashmere sweaters instead of just one, call up your high-school sweetheart just to say "hi," and start eating dessert first.

Life is too short to be subtle. Carry on!

Inner Strength Builds

You have been tested, and you have passed. Maybe it wasn't always pretty; maybe you didn't always get the highest grade. So what? At this point, after cancer, you are no stranger to adversity. You know what you can ask of yourself, and you know what you're made of.

Surviving cancer is no little accomplishment. The inner strength that you developed during the course of treatment will continue to grow.

People Matter More

One day over lunch, a man we know confided that before he started treatments for cancer, eating lunch with a friend was no big deal — it was just a break in the middle of the workday. "Now," he said earnestly, "having lunch with someone whose company I enjoy feels like a privilege, a special occasion."

He was right. After cancer, close personal relationships take on extra meaning. Even unexpected conversations with people you don't know well somehow seem more significant, more interesting than before. You likely will seek out connections with others.

Forgiveness Gains in Importance

You say you used to be a pro at holding a grudge? Don't be surprised if that changes right along with your perspective on what matters in life. Maybe it never mattered before that you didn't get along with your in-laws or your sister's husband's daughter or your neighbor. Cancer has a way of making most people more mellow, more willing to look at the big picture, more willing to let bygones be bygones.

If you were compassionate before, now you may be more so. If, from time to time, you were thankful for all the good things in your life, now you may live in a continuous state of gratitude. If previously you looked for the good in people, now you will point out their sterling qualities to anyone who will listen.

Being grateful to be alive does not mean taking whatever others dole out, and it does not preclude sticking up for yourself when you are wronged. You need not have a full-blown tantrum, of course, but by all means point out the transgression — then move on.

On the other hand, maybe you used to be a crotchety curmudgeon — and proud of it — and after cancer you're sticking to that personality. Far be it for us to insist on personal transformations that don't feel natural!

Support Comes Naturally

During this period when you realize more acutely than ever that people who need people are the luckiest people in the world, you may find that you are eager to comfort a friend facing an illness, even if you have not been close friends before. When you get the e-mail at work that says a colleague has been diagnosed with cancer, you may find yourself jotting down the address and putting a card in the mail.

In a way, you speak a new language after cancer. More than ever, you know what words to say to encourage someone else. Even if you never felt comfortable saying them before, you'll say them now.

The Tongue Loosens

About this new language: Often, after cancer, you may feel compelled to express your appreciation more freely, speak of your personal allegiances more openly, and even proclaim your love more readily.

Yikes! What's that about?

Go back and read the section "A Sense of Adventure Grows." This new tendency to express your emotions likely is a direct result of the realization that life is, indeed, too short to be subtle or to be shy or to not say what needs to be said when it needs to be said. So speak up!

Time Flies

One minute, you look in the mirror and decide your hair is long enough to go out without your wig, and the next, you clearly need to make an appointment to get your hair cut.

One day, the trees are budding out and the days are growing longer, and before you know it the summer months have slipped by and you are on the downhill slide to the turkey.

One month, you've saved enough to replace that old couch in the den where you used to nap during chemo, and in a few short years, your grandchildren have spilled so much juice and goodness-knows-what-else on the "new" couch that you realize you need slipcovers — or another new couch.

One year, you invite a half-dozen close friends, members of your support team, to join you for dinner as you mark the fifth anniversary of your cancer diagnosis. Dinner is barely over, or so it seems, when you're treating yourself to a trip to Italy to celebrate the ninth anniversary of that diagnosis.

What happened?

Time flies. It always has, but after cancer, you treasure the time you have and carefully make the most of it.

Chapter 25

Ten Sources for More Information

In This Chapter

▶ Finding resources online

▶ Picking up a magazine

*W*here do you go for additional information on cancer? In a word, everywhere. For starters, your doctors likely can provide you with free booklets on cancer-related topics that directly affect you, and bookstores stock shelves full of titles that deal with cancer. Don't forget to look at your local library, as well.

All the major cancer agencies have Web sites on the Internet, and you can also find assorted news groups, e-mail lists, and online newsletters. We also know of one magazine published specifically for people living with cancer. In this chapter, we get you started tracking down some of the available resources.

Searching the Web

A word of caution is an order about information on the Internet. Some of it comes from reliable sources. Some of it comes from companies looking to make a profit from products said to help people with cancer. Some of it shows up on individuals' home pages, perhaps as a recounting of personal experiences with cancer.

Any and all of these sites may offer something of value, but if you are specifically interested in scientifically accurate information, look for the logo of the Health on the Net Foundation. This international organization based in Switzerland reviews medical and health-related information on the Web and awards its logo to those that fulfill stringent requirements regarding medical content.

Following are some particularly useful sources of information on the Internet.

National Cancer Institute

The National Cancer Institute (NCI) is part of the federal government's National Institutes of Health. The Web site — www.nci.nih.gov — provides information in English and Spanish on types of cancer, types of treatments, clinical trials, cancer statistics, and news reports on cancer research.

The Web site also lists free NCI publications on types of cancer, treatment options, clinical trials, nutrition, and other topics. You have three options:

- Download the information.
- Print an order form and mail it in.
- Call to order the booklets.

The number for the Cancer Information Service at NCI is 1-800-4-CANCER (1-800-422-6237).

American Cancer Society

This agency's Web site — at www.cancer.org — offers information on types of cancer, clinical trials, treatment options, and coping strategies, as well as "news you can use." Information is available in Spanish, and some materials are available in Asian languages. The site's bookstore offers a variety of books on different aspects of cancer and health.

The site also has a Cancer Survivors Network, message boards, and a service that provides information on programs and activities available through the American Cancer Society office in or near your hometown. You may also call 1-800-ACS-2345 (1-800-227-2345).

National Comprehensive Cancer Network

The National Comprehensive Cancer Network (NCCN) — on the Web at www.nccn.org — is an alliance of 19 cancer centers located around the world that serves as a resource for oncologists and people with cancer. A not-for-profit organization, the NCCN develops guidelines that are the standard for clinical policy in oncology. If you click on Patients and then on Patient Guidelines, you find information on treatments for various types of cancer, provided in English and Spanish.

American Society for Therapeutic Radiology and Oncology

Known as ASTRO, this professional radiation oncology association is dedicated to improving patient care through education and the advancement of science. On the Web site — www.astro.org — click on <u>Patients</u> and then on <u>Treatment Information</u>. There, seven booklets are available on radiation therapy for different types of cancer. You may download them or send an e-mail to carolc@astro.org to request a copy. You also may type in your city to locate the name of a radiation oncologist near you.

People Living With Cancer

The American Society of Clinical Oncology (ASCO) maintains this Web site — at www.plwc.org — where ASCO provides information on more than 50 different types of cancer and respective treatments, clinical trials, coping strategies, and side effects. The site also offers a list of ASCO-affiliated oncologists, live chats, message boards, and links to support organizations.

OncoLink

Billed as "the Web's first cancer resource," the Abramson Cancer Center of the University of Pennsylvania Web site — at www.oncolink.upenn.edu — offers information on types of cancer, treatment options, and clinical trials, plus news reports, a tip of the day, and a monthly e-newsletter.

Planet Cancer

Of the many Web sites for cancer survivors, this one — at www.planet cancer.org — targets young adults "between pediatric and geriatric." Founded by three young survivors in Austin, Texas, the site offers comics, stories, tips, and information on gatherings around the country for young adults who have survived cancer.

Coalition of National Cancer Cooperative Groups

This organization offers TrialCheck, which provides nationwide locations for clinical trials that are open and enrolling patients. The site — at www.trial check.org — also offers general information about clinical trials for anyone considering participating.

National Marrow Donor Program

Based in Minneapolis, this nonprofit organization is a consortium of more than 150 medical centers located across the country that specialize in bone marrow and stem cell transplants. For a state-by-state list of centers affiliated with the National Marrow Donor Program, call 888-999-6743 or see www.marrow.org. At the Web site, click on Patient Resources.

The organization also maintains an international registry of potential donors for all sources of blood stem cells used in transplantation. See www.marrow. org or call 800-627-7692 for more information.

Coping with Cancer Magazine

Now in its 18th year, the magazine *Coping with Cancer* counts among its readers people with cancer, their families, caregivers, healthcare teams, and support group leaders. In fact, you may see copies of the magazine at your doctor's office or at your local branch of The Wellness Community.

To subscribe, you may call 615-791-3859 or sign up at www.copingmag.com. A one-year subscription (six issues) costs $19.

Glossary

 n this glossary, we provide brief definitions for many of the medical and technical terms used in the book. Though many of these terms are defined in detail within the text, we offer this handy list so you can refer back to something that you read or heard your doctor say.

adrenalectomy: Surgical removal of the adrenal gland.

allogeneic transplant: A transplant in which you receive stem cells from a relative or an unrelated donor.

alopecia: Hair loss.

alternative therapies: Therapies — generally untested — that are used in place of chemotherapy or radiation treatments.

anemia: A lack of red blood cells that leads to fatigue, weakness, and shortness of breath.

anesthesia: Medications or gases that cause a lack of feeling or numbness.

anorexia: Loss of appetite.

antibodies: Part of the body's defense system against bacteria or blood cells.

antigen: A substance that triggers production of an antibody.

asanas: Postures or poses in yoga.

autologous transplant: A transplant in which you receive your own stem cells.

benign tumor: A noncancerous tumor.

bias: An effect on the result of a clinical trial caused by personal choices.

biological therapy: Treatment that stimulates or restores the functioning of the immune system.

biopsy: The removal of cells or tissue for medical examination.

blood cell count: A rating of the number of red blood cells, white blood cells, and platelets in any given blood sample.

bone marrow: Spongy tissue inside bones where blood cells are manufactured.

bone marrow transplant: A procedure that replaces bone marrow that is purposely destroyed by high doses of cancer drugs or radiation.

bone scan: An imaging test to determine whether cancer has spread.

brachytherapy: Internal radiation therapy using seeds or wires filled with radioactive materials.

cachexia: Wasting syndrome, which leads to loss of weight, fat, and muscle.

cancer: A word used to describe more than 100 diseases that all involve abnormal cell growth.

carcinogen: A substance that causes cancer.

carcinoma: Cancer that develops in tissues covering or lining organs of the body.

catheter: A flexible tube used to deliver anticancer drugs into the body.

chemotherapy: Treatment with anticancer drugs.

clinical trial: A scientific study that evaluates new treatments or combinations of treatments.

colony stimulating factor: A substance that stimulates the production of blood cells.

complementary therapies: Nonmedical therapies, such as yoga or tai chi, that are often recommended to relieve stress while undergoing cancer treatments.

computer-assisted tomography: Detailed pictures of the inside of the body made by a computer linked to an x-ray machine; also known as a _CT scan_.

cryopreservation: A storage process for biological material in which the material of interest is frozen.

diuretic: Medication that increases urine output.

DNA: Deoxyribonucleic acid, which carries genetic material in the body.

endocrine system: Glands that regulate bodily functions.

endoscopy: A screening test to examine the inside of the body.

engraftment: A process in which transplanted cells begin to produce new white blood cells, red blood cells, and platelets.

enteral therapy: Feeding through a tube into the stomach or intestine.

erythrocytes: Red blood cells.

external beam radiation: Radiation therapy that aims high-energy rays at a tumor or a site where a tumor was removed.

flavonoid: Plant pigments in food thought to protect the body from cancer.

gene therapy: The manipulation of genetic material to treat disease.

grade: A ranking (1 through 4) of the degree to which malignant cells resemble healthy cells.

growth factor: See *colony stimulating factor.*

hematopoiesis: The formation and development of blood cells.

Hippocrates: A Greek physician who lived in the fifth century B.C. and gave his name to the famous oath that physicians take upon graduation from medical school.

hospice care: Compassionate end-of-life care proved in the home, hospital, or nursing home.

hypophysectomy: Surgical removal of the pituitary gland.

immune system: A complex group of organs and cells that defend the body against disease.

infertility: The inability to conceive or to carry a fetus to term.

intercellular: Located between cells.

intravenous: Injected into a blood vessel.

leukocytes: White blood cells.

leukopenia: A low level of white blood cells; also called *neutropenia.*

linear accelerator: A machine that delivers external beam radiation treatment.

lymphatic system: Tissues and organs that produce, store, and transport white blood cells throughout the body.

lymphedema: Swelling caused by lymphatic fluids that collect in tissues.

lymphoma: Cancer in cells of the lymphatic system.

macrophage: A white blood cell that devours and digests viruses.

magnetic resonance imaging: A scan in which a magnet linked to a computer creates detailed pictures of the inside of the body; also known as an _MRI_.

malignant tumor: A cancerous tumor.

medical oncologist: A medical specialist who treats cancer.

metastasis: The spread of cancer from one organ or part of the body to another.

mutation: A change in the structure of a gene that may lead to cancer.

oophorectomy: Surgical removal of the ovaries.

orchiectomy: Surgical removal of the testicles; also known as _surgical castration_.

ostomy: An excretory opening constructed surgically.

Pap test: A screening test for cervical cancer.

parenteral nutrition: Feeding through the bloodstream.

pharmacopeia: A compilation of pharmaceutical products.

phytoestrogens: Natural plant compounds that act like estrogen in the body.

platelets: Blood cells that help blood to clot.

pneumonitis: Inflammation and/or infection of lung tissue; also known as _pneumonia_.

prognosis: A likely outcome or chance for recovery from a disease.

protocol: The action plan for a clinical trial.

radiation oncologist: A medical doctor who treats cancer patients with radiation therapy.

radiation "recall": Continued skin sensitivity after radiation treatments have ended.

radiation tattoos: Marks made on the skin with India ink or marking pens that map the area to be treated.

recurrence: The return of cancer after it had disappeared.

reiki: A form of body work often used as a complementary healing practice.

remission: A time period when signs and symptoms of cancer disappear.

restorative yoga: A style of yoga where participants lie on the floor, supported by bolsters and blankets, and concentrate on relaxation.

retrieval: A procedure in which stem cells are removed from a donor.

RNA: Ribonucleic acid, which controls the synthesis of new proteins after transcribing genetic information from DNA.

side effects: Health problems that result from cancer treatments.

spiritual distress: Guilt, a loss of faith, or a sudden feeling that life has no meaning.

stage: The extent of cancer determined to be in the body.

staging: The purpose of tests and scans that determine the extent of cancer in the body.

stem cells: Primitive cells in marrow that help make red blood cells, white blood cells, and platelets.

syngeneic transplant: A transplant in which stem cells are transplanted from an identical twin.

systemic: Treatment that affects cells throughout the body.

tai chi: An ancient Chinese practice that features a series of sustained, flowing movements.

T cell: A type of white blood cell that works to destroy viruses.

therapeutic massage: A form of body work often used as a complementary therapy.

thrombocytes: Platelets, which help blood to clot.

thrombocytopenia: A low platelet count.

Transcendental Meditation: A form of deep relaxation often used as a complementary therapy.

transfusion: A medical treatment designed to build up blood cell counts.

tryptophan: A chemical found in chocolate (and turkey) that the brain uses to make serotonin, which in turn produces feelings of joy and well-being.

tumor: A mass of tissue that results from abnormal, excessive cell division. Some tumors are cancerous; others are not.

ultrasonography: A screening test in which ultrasound (sound waves) is bounced off tissues and the echoes are converted into a picture.

Index

• K •

• *T* •

BUSINESS, CAREERS & PERSONAL FINANCE

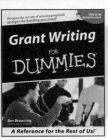

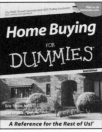

0-7645-5307-0   0-7645-5331-3 *†

Also available:
- Accounting For Dummies †
  0-7645-5314-3
- Business Plans Kit For Dummies †
  0-7645-5365-8
- Cover Letters For Dummies
  0-7645-5224-4
- Frugal Living For Dummies
  0-7645-5403-4
- Leadership For Dummies
  0-7645-5176-0
- Managing For Dummies
  0-7645-1771-6

- Marketing For Dummies
  0-7645-5600-2
- Personal Finance For Dummies *
  0-7645-2590-5
- Project Management For Dummies
  0-7645-5283-X
- Resumes For Dummies †
  0-7645-5471-9
- Selling For Dummies
  0-7645-5363-1
- Small Business Kit For Dummies *†
  0-7645-5093-4

HOME & BUSINESS COMPUTER BASICS

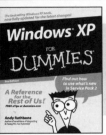

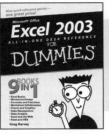

0-7645-4074-2   0-7645-3758-X

Also available:
- ACT! 6 For Dummies
  0-7645-2645-6
- iLife '04 All-in-One Desk Reference
  For Dummies
  0-7645-7347-0
- iPAQ For Dummies
  0-7645-6769-1
- Mac OS X Panther Timesaving
  Techniques For Dummies
  0-7645-5812-9
- Macs For Dummies
  0-7645-5656-8

- Microsoft Money 2004 For Dummies
  0-7645-4195-1
- Office 2003 All-in-One Desk Reference
  For Dummies
  0-7645-3883-7
- Outlook 2003 For Dummies
  0-7645-3759-8
- PCs For Dummies
  0-7645-4074-2
- TiVo For Dummies
  0-7645-6923-6
- Upgrading and Fixing PCs For Dummies
  0-7645-1665-5
- Windows XP Timesaving Techniques
  For Dummies
  0-7645-3748-2

FOOD, HOME, GARDEN, HOBBIES, MUSIC & PETS

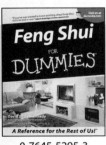

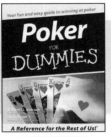

0-7645-5295-3   0-7645-5232-5

Also available:
- Bass Guitar For Dummies
  0-7645-2487-9
- Diabetes Cookbook For Dummies
  0-7645-5230-9
- Gardening For Dummies *
  0-7645-5130-2
- Guitar For Dummies
  0-7645-5106-X
- Holiday Decorating For Dummies
  0-7645-2570-0
- Home Improvement All-in-One
  For Dummies
  0-7645-5680-0

- Knitting For Dummies
  0-7645-5395-X
- Piano For Dummies
  0-7645-5105-1
- Puppies For Dummies
  0-7645-5255-4
- Scrapbooking For Dummies
  0-7645-7208-3
- Senior Dogs For Dummies
  0-7645-5818-8
- Singing For Dummies
  0-7645-2475-5
- 30-Minute Meals For Dummies
  0-7645-2589-1

INTERNET & DIGITAL MEDIA

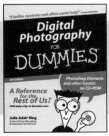

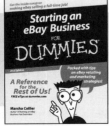

0-7645-1664-7   0-7645-6924-4

Also available:
- 2005 Online Shopping Directory
  For Dummies
  0-7645-7495-7
- CD & DVD Recording For Dummies
  0-7645-5956-7
- eBay For Dummies
  0-7645-5654-1
- Fighting Spam For Dummies
  0-7645-5965-6
- Genealogy Online For Dummies
  0-7645-5964-8
- Google For Dummies
  0-7645-4420-9

- Home Recording For Musicians
  For Dummies
  0-7645-1634-5
- The Internet For Dummies
  0-7645-4173-0
- iPod & iTunes For Dummies
  0-7645-7772-7
- Preventing Identity Theft For Dummies
  0-7645-7336-5
- Pro Tools All-in-One Desk Reference
  For Dummies
  0-7645-5714-9
- Roxio Easy Media Creator For Dummies
  0-7645-7131-1

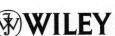 **WILEY**

SPORTS, FITNESS, PARENTING, RELIGION & SPIRITUALITY

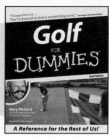

0-7645-5146-9

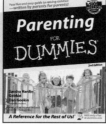

0-7645-5418-2

Also available:

✔ Adoption For Dummies
0-7645-5488-3

✔ Basketball For Dummies
0-7645-5248-1

✔ The Bible For Dummies
0-7645-5296-1

✔ Buddhism For Dummies
0-7645-5359-3

✔ Catholicism For Dummies
0-7645-5391-7

✔ Hockey For Dummies
0-7645-5228-7

✔ Judaism For Dummies
0-7645-5299-6

✔ Martial Arts For Dummies
0-7645-5358-5

✔ Pilates For Dummies
0-7645-5397-6

✔ Religion For Dummies
0-7645-5264-3

✔ Teaching Kids to Read For Dummies
0-7645-4043-2

✔ Weight Training For Dummies
0-7645-5168-X

✔ Yoga For Dummies
0-7645-5117-5

TRAVEL

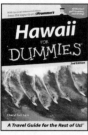

0-7645-5438-7

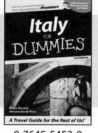

0-7645-5453-0

Also available:

✔ Alaska For Dummies
0-7645-1761-9

✔ Arizona For Dummies
0-7645-6938-4

✔ Cancún and the Yucatán For Dummies
0-7645-2437-2

✔ Cruise Vacations For Dummies
0-7645-6941-4

✔ Europe For Dummies
0-7645-5456-5

✔ Ireland For Dummies
0-7645-5455-7

✔ Las Vegas For Dummies
0-7645-5448-4

✔ London For Dummies
0-7645-4277-X

✔ New York City For Dummies
0-7645-6945-7

✔ Paris For Dummies
0-7645-5494-8

✔ RV Vacations For Dummies
0-7645-5443-3

✔ Walt Disney World & Orlando For Dummies
0-7645-6943-0

GRAPHICS, DESIGN & WEB DEVELOPMENT

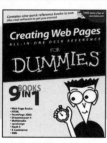

0-7645-4345-8

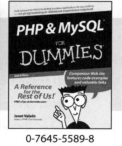

0-7645-5589-8

Also available:

✔ Adobe Acrobat 6 PDF For Dummies
0-7645-3760-1

✔ Building a Web Site For Dummies
0-7645-7144-3

✔ Dreamweaver MX 2004 For Dummies
0-7645-4342-3

✔ FrontPage 2003 For Dummies
0-7645-3882-9

✔ HTML 4 For Dummies
0-7645-1995-6

✔ Illustrator cs For Dummies
0-7645-4084-X

✔ Macromedia Flash MX 2004 For Dummies
0-7645-4358-X

✔ Photoshop 7 All-in-One Desk Reference For Dummies
0-7645-1667-1

✔ Photoshop cs Timesaving Techniques For Dummies
0-7645-6782-9

✔ PHP 5 For Dummies
0-7645-4166-8

✔ PowerPoint 2003 For Dummies
0-7645-3908-6

✔ QuarkXPress 6 For Dummies
0-7645-2593-X

NETWORKING, SECURITY, PROGRAMMING & DATABASES

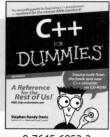

0-7645-6852-3

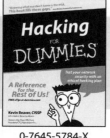

0-7645-5784-X

Also available:

✔ A+ Certification For Dummies
0-7645-4187-0

✔ Access 2003 All-in-One Desk Reference For Dummies
0-7645-3988-4

✔ Beginning Programming For Dummies
0-7645-4997-9

✔ C For Dummies
0-7645-7068-4

✔ Firewalls For Dummies
0-7645-4048-3

✔ Home Networking For Dummies
0-7645-42796

✔ Network Security For Dummies
0-7645-1679-5

✔ Networking For Dummies
0-7645-1677-9

✔ TCP/IP For Dummies
0-7645-1760-0

✔ VBA For Dummies
0-7645-3989-2

✔ Wireless All In-One Desk Reference For Dummies
0-7645-7496-5

✔ Wireless Home Networking For Dummies
0-7645-3910-8

HEALTH & SELF-HELP

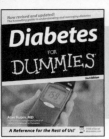
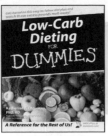

0-7645-6820-5 *†

0-7645-2566-2

Also available:
- Alzheimer's For Dummies
  0-7645-3899-3
- Asthma For Dummies
  0-7645-4233-8
- Controlling Cholesterol For Dummies
  0-7645-5440-9
- Depression For Dummies
  0-7645-3900-0
- Dieting For Dummies
  0-7645-4149-8
- Fertility For Dummies
  0-7645-2549-2

- Fibromyalgia For Dummies
  0-7645-5441-7
- Improving Your Memory For Dummies
  0-7645-5435-2
- Pregnancy For Dummies †
  0-7645-4483-7
- Quitting Smoking For Dummies
  0-7645-2629-4
- Relationships For Dummies
  0-7645-5384-4
- Thyroid For Dummies
  0-7645-5385-2

EDUCATION, HISTORY, REFERENCE & TEST PREPARATION

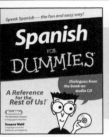
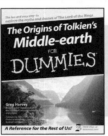

0-7645-5194-9

0-7645-4186-2

Also available:
- Algebra For Dummies
  0-7645-5325-9
- British History For Dummies
  0-7645-7021-8
- Calculus For Dummies
  0-7645-2498-4
- English Grammar For Dummies
  0-7645-5322-4
- Forensics For Dummies
  0-7645-5580-4
- The GMAT For Dummies
  0-7645-5251-1
- Inglés Para Dummies
  0-7645-5427-1

- Italian For Dummies
  0-7645-5196-5
- Latin For Dummies
  0-7645-5431-X
- Lewis & Clark For Dummies
  0-7645-2545-X
- Research Papers For Dummies
  0-7645-5426-3
- The SAT I For Dummies
  0-7645-7193-1
- Science Fair Projects For Dummies
  0-7645-5460-3
- U.S. History For Dummies
  0-7645-5249-X

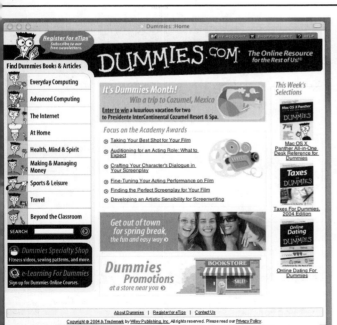

Get smart @ dummies.com®

- **Find a full list of Dummies titles**
- **Look into loads of FREE on-site articles**
- **Sign up for FREE eTips e-mailed to you weekly**
- **See what other products carry the Dummies name**
- **Shop directly from the Dummies bookstore**
- **Enter to win new prizes every month!**

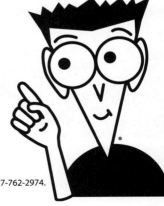

* Separate Canadian edition also available
† Separate U.K. edition also available

Available wherever books are sold. For more information or to order direct: U.S. customers visit www.dummies.com or call 1-877-762-2974.
U.K. customers visit www.wileyeurope.com or call 0800 243407. Canadian customers visit www.wiley.ca or call 1-800-567-4797.

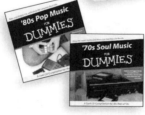
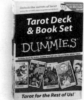
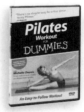
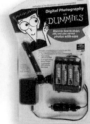
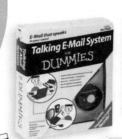
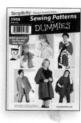
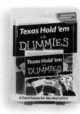
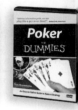
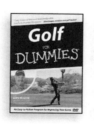
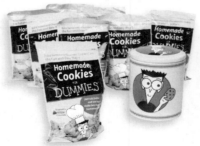
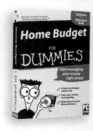
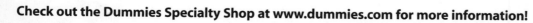
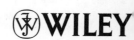